TECHNOLOGICAL MEDICINE

The Changing World of Doctors and Patients

Advances in medicine have brought us the stethoscope, artificial kidneys, and computerized health records. They have also changed the doctor-patient relationship.

This book explores how the technologies of medicine are created and how we respond to the problems and successes of their use. Stanley Joel Reiser, MD, walks us through the ways medical innovations exert their influence by discussing a number of selected technologies including the X-ray, ultrasound, and respirator. Reiser creates a new understanding of thinking about how health care is practiced in the United States and thereby suggests new approaches to effectively meet the challenges of living with technological medicine.

As health care reform continues to be an intensely debated topic in America, *Technological Medicine* shows us the pros and cons of applying technological solutions to health and illness.

Stanley Joel Reiser, Clinical Professor of Health Care Sciences and of Health Policy at The George Washington University School of Medicine and Health Sciences, is known nationally and internationally for his scholarship and teaching in ethics, history, technology assessment, and health policy. Before arriving at The George Washington University, he held teaching positions at Harvard University and the University of Texas Health Science Center at Houston. He has written more than 120 books and essays. His articles have appeared in such publications as *Journal of the American Medical Association, New England Journal of Medicine, Annals of Internal Medicine, American Journal of Public Health, Health Affairs, Hastings Center Report, Scientific American,* and *The New York Times.*

TECHNOLOGICAL MEDICINE

The Changing World of Doctors and Patients

———

STANLEY JOEL REISER

The George Washington University School of Medicine and Health Sciences

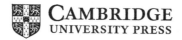

CAMBRIDGE
UNIVERSITY PRESS

32 Avenue of the Americas, New York NY 10013-2473, USA

Cambridge University Press is part of the University of Cambridge.

It furthers the University's mission by disseminating knowledge in the pursuit of education, learning and research at the highest international levels of excellence.

www.cambridge.org
Information on this title: www.cambridge.org/9781107661233

© Stanley Joel Reiser 2009

First published 2009
First paperback edition 2014

A catalogue record for this publication is available from the British Library

Library of Congress Cataloguing in Publication data
Reiser, Stanley Joel.
Technological medicine : the changing world of doctors and patients /
Stanley Joel Reiser.
p. ; cm.
Includes bibliographical references and index.
ISBN 978-0-521-83569-5 (hardback)
1. Medical innovations.   2. Medical technology.   I. Title.
[DNLM: 1. Biomedical Technology – trends.   2. Biomedical Technology – history.
3. History, Modern 1601–.   W 82 R377e 2009]
RA418.5.M4.R45   2009
610.28'4 – dc22   2009010914

ISBN 978-0-521-83569-5 Hardback
ISBN 978-1-107-66123-3 Paperback

*Remembering: Sylvia and Harry Reiser
and I. Bernard Cohen*

*Celebrating: Katharyn, Traci, Adam, Vanessa,
Thomas, Caroline, and Tessa*

CONTENTS

LIST OF ILLUSTRATIONS

LIST OF TABLES

PREFACE

This book explores how the technologies of medicine are created; how society, patients, and practitioners respond to the problems and successes of their use; and how this response changes them. For as we create technology and strive to apply its powers, it re-creates us. To demonstrate the different ways through which medical innovations exert their influence, a number of selected technologies are examined. We explore how the first widely used technology to diagnose illness, the stethoscope, transformed the relationship between patients and doctors as it revealed hidden sounds produced in us by disease. We probe the elation and benefits experienced by doctors and the public when the X-ray gave them the power to see into the body and the unanticipated problems its use created. We examine the creation of the artificial kidney and the public efforts first to ration its use and then to fund it. The development of the artificial respirator and a journey that led it to sustain polio victims and later irreversibly comatose patients is explored, with its generation of medical, legal, and ethical quandaries. The events leading to the electronic health record, hailed in contemporary times by doctors, policy makers, and the public as a key to a less costly and more effective health system are probed and the promises of this belief examined. This is followed by considering the rise of scientific means to determine whether therapies are effective or not, such as the randomized clinical trial; and the innovative social and medical decision process Oregon instituted to decide what therapies to offer through publicly funded programs. Technologies to prevent disease and the ambiguous place of securing health as a goal of medical practice are probed, after which the transformation of birth from a social to a technologically driven medical event is discussed, followed by an explanation of the nature of technology and how it exerts its compelling influence. The understandings gained from this exploration are then applied to suggest fundamental ways to change thinking and practice in health care, and thereby to meet more effectively the challenges of using and living with technological medicine. The book is written for a public, health professional, and health policy readership.

In developing the content for and in writing this book, I have had the constant support and insightful criticism of its editor at Cambridge University Press, Richard L. Ziemacki, to whom I am deeply grateful. In guiding the book through later stages of editing and production, Cambridge editor Eric Crahan made creative and valued contributions, and Shana Meyer, project manager at Aptara Inc., provided always perceptive suggestions.

Securing the literature and illustrations for the work was furthered greatly by the gracious assistance and informative suggestions of the staff of the Himmelfarb Health Sciences Library at The George Washington University Medical Center, among whom I am particularly indebted to Cynthia Kahn, whose bibliographical and historical expertise and timely help greatly furthered my research. The history librarian at the American College of Obstetricians and Gynecologists, Deborah Scarborough, gave me invaluable access to its extensive historical works. I received similarly gracious help from the staff of the National Museum of Health and Medicine of the Armed Forces Institute of Pathology: James Curley and Alan Hawk from its Historical Collections division, and Michael Rhode at the museum's Otis Historical Archives. The holdings of the National Library of Medicine were opened to me by its knowledgeable and always-helpful staff: Stephen Greenberg provided astute analysis of bibliographical issues, and Crystal Smith important assistance in securing documents and literature; Paul Thierman and Sara Eilers gave me expert guidance in finding excellent illustrations. These and other visual material for the book were electronically retrieved and formatted by Robert K. Foreman at the Computer Application and Support Services of The George Washington University Medical Center, for whose insightful work with this material I am most appreciative.

A number of individuals read and criticized different chapters in the book and offered helpful suggestions on aspects of my work. For this, I gratefully acknowledge the late Clifford Dancer, the late Ruth Luzzati, Mark Novitch, Adam Harry Reiser, and Vanessa Reiser Shaw.

The book was begun at the University of Texas Health Science Center at Houston, and I am especially indebted to Janice Glover, John Porretto, and R. Palmer Beasley for their important help with this effort. In 2005 I was invited to be the James Clark Welling Visiting Professor at The George Washington University School of Medicine and Health Sciences, and I made periodic visits to lecture at the university during the next two years. In 2007 I moved to Washington, D.C., to join the medical school faculty, and I completed a large portion of the book under the stimulus of its vibrant and humanistic environment. I am grateful to Stephen Joel Trachtenberg, James C. Scott, and W. Scott Schroth both for the initial opportunity to teach there and for their continued encouragement of my work.

Finally, my wife, Katharyn Dancer Reiser, provided support at all levels of the manuscript's development. Her presence pervades the pages of this book, which could not have been written without her devoted concern and effort.

Stanley Joel Reiser
Washington, D.C.
January 2009

REVEALING THE BODY'S WHISPERS

How the Stethoscope Transformed Medicine

"Technological breakthrough" is a phrase that stirs visions of a complex invention having multiple parts that do something important. In medicine we think of artificial hearts, respirators, and imaging machines. But sometimes the material expression of a significant concept appears in a plain wrapper. No technology illustrates this more than a wooden tube with an opening down the center created in 1816 by the French physician René Laennec, which revolutionized diagnosis, altered the doctor's identity, transformed the experience of being a patient, and changed medicine forever. He called it the stethoscope.

The transformative power of this tube had as much to do with its effects on the relationship between doctor and patient as it did with the evidence of illness that it uncovered. In medicine, relationships and evidence are linked. How the facts about an illness are gathered and the nature of those facts critically affect how doctor and patient regard each other. The influence of technology on these connections is demonstrated by the story of the stethoscope's invention and use. But to set the stage for its coming, we need to explore earlier means used by doctors to investigate medical problems.

Before stethoscopes, the coin of evaluation was words – the doctor learned about an illness from the patient's story of the events and sensations marking its passage. Patient-driven narratives appear in early works of Western medicine, such as those written by Hippocrates and his disciples in ancient Greece more than two and a half millennia ago. One case begins: "Silenus lived on Broadway, near the place of Eualcidas. After over-exertion, drinking, and exercises at the wrong time he was attacked by fever. He began having pains in the loins, with heaviness in the head and tightness in the neck. From the bowels on the first day there passed copious discharges of bilious matter, unmixed, frothy, and highly coloured. Urine black, with a black sediment; thirst; tongue dry; no sleep at night."[1] Most of the symptoms described in the case were felt or witnessed by the patient and transmitted to the doctor. The case report continued until the eleventh day of the illness, when Silenus died.

More than two thousand years later, in the seventeenth century, the narrative account of illness by patients was still the main way that the doctor obtained facts on which to base a diagnosis and suggest a remedy. It did not matter whether the narrative was given by the patient in person or sent by mail to the doctor for a written opinion. In fact, the practice of consultation by letter was widespread at the time, an index of the significance of the patient's narrative. A doctor of the period often consulted in this way was John Symcotts, an English physician with a large practice in Huntington and Bedfordshire and for many years physician to Oliver Cromwell and his family. He got the following request for help by mail:

Sir,

I have a great burning pain about the reins of my back, which strikes up to the top of my belly, and a wonderful ill scent arising from my stomach. I do desire your best advice. In my hankering for physic I have taken so much all ready and it has done me no good, and therefore I would desire you to send me no physic but some oil or some cooling thing, for I am very sore about my back that I cannot stand upright. The greatest pain of all is my left kidney.[2]

The focus of the stories is the illness as experienced by and depicted through the feelings and words of the patient. The patient as sufferer held center stage: the patient was the narrator of the illness as well as its victim, and the doctor's decisions about what was needed were largely determined by what the patient said. The doctor's success or failure with the remedies prescribed was also measured by the patient's view of their effects. The doctor was brought into the patient's life and world of remembrance. There the doctor resided throughout the illness, as so much hung on the patient's view.

This position was not always comfortable for doctors. For example, William Cullen, professor of medicine at schools in Glasgow and Edinburgh, wrote in his 1789 treatise on the classification of diseases that he always preferred symptoms "perceived by the physician, rather than by the patient, yet the latter, however fallacious, are not wholly to be rejected."[3] Another well-known physician and professor of anatomy at Edinburgh, Alexander Monro, commented in an 1811 book that the story patients gave of their illnesses was flawed in several ways, such as "the imperfect manner in which patients describe their ailments, and the erroneous account which many physicians lead their patients to give of their situation, from taking up too hasty an opinion respecting the nature of the case."[4] Monro grasped the problem that physicians dependent on the story of patients faced: usually there was no good way to judge the accuracy of the patient's recollections. But he also recognized that, knowingly or unwittingly, doctors might influence the patient's narrative to reflect their own views about what was the matter.

Physicians like Cullen and Monro did have means of exploring illness other than accepting the patient's perspective: they could see and touch the body. When exploring the patient's outward appearance, doctors focused on facial expression, posture, gait, and the tongue. They looked also at matter generated from within, such as urine, stools, and gastric matter, and blood, when it was expelled from the body or deliberately let out for therapeutic purposes.

However, doctors exercised restraint in examining the body physically and limited their inquiries largely to evaluating the pulse, body heat, and tumorous outgrowths emerging at the surface of the skin. Physicians had eschewed deep probing with the hands or using instruments to examine the body ever since the study of medicine had been placed in universities in the thirteenth century. The university-trained physicians considered active manipulation of the body or use of instruments on it to be menial actions beneath their station as learned professionals and best left to healers of lower status. The training of physicians in these universities followed the same scholastic and text-driven approach to learning used to teach theology and law, the two other main branches of university education. So in this environment, theoretical exploration and discourse, not hands-on practical knowledge seeking, reigned supreme. This perspective determined the doctor's approach to practice. Accordingly, physicians mainly listened to stories of patients, inspected their appearance, and gently explored the body's surface to decide what was wrong.

The revolution that changed how doctors learned about illness and related to patients, and reversed their attitudes about actively exploring the body and using tools, began with and was vitally nourished by the study of the dead. Many controversies about how the body was put together and what its architecture really looked like were resolved with the appearance of the 1543 work on anatomy by Andreas Vesalius, *De humani corporis fabrica*, which for the first time gave doctors a detailed picture of every major part of the body.[5] The work facilitated the study of the normal composition of the body and, critically, spurred the investigation of structural changes created by disease in it through the emerging discipline of pathology.

The equivalent for pathology of Vesalius's work appeared two centuries later when Giovanni Battista Morgagni published in 1761 *The Seats and Causes of Diseases Investigated by Anatomy*.[6] Its title described its theme. Morgagni showed that the footprints of different illnesses could be recognized in characteristic disruptions they created in the body's inner architecture. Further, he demonstrated that these disruptions of structure, or lesions, directly caused the expressions of illness displayed in the living person called symptoms. Morgagni's work and ideas have defined the basic way physicians think about illness from the time of his book's publication to the present. This way of understanding disease is centered on one question: where is the disease? An anatomical view of illness requires locating its presence in some place in the body. As the title of Morgagni's work describes, diseases have seats in the body. Locate the seat and you explain both the origin of the illness and the reasons a patient has particular symptoms.

But the concept raised a fascinating problem for doctors. How to locate the lesions beneath the skin of a living patient without piercing it with a scalpel? What good was anatomical thinking without a dependable, noninvasive way of finding the lesions in patients? Clinicians began to appreciate that something more precise than the verbal accounts of patients or the outer survey of the body was needed to take full advantage of the new anatomical insights. From the publication of Morgagni's book, fifty-five years would pass before a generic solution to this problem appeared. The answer would emerge from what had started as an ordinary clinical consultation.

In 1816 a thirty-five-year-old French doctor, René Laennec, was consulted at the Necker Hospital in Paris by a young woman with symptoms of heart disease. To probe her illness, Laennec thought of a technique first suggested by Hippocrates, who urged physicians to put their ear on their patient's chest to determine whether water (which would sound like boiling vinegar) or pus was present. This technique, called auscultation, had been largely ignored. However, Laennec and his medical colleague, Gaspard Bayle, occasionally used it, particularly to evaluate heartbeats. But it required doctors to move their head over the surface of the patient's body, a procedure not only cumbersome and unpleasant to both but also, when doctor and patient did not share a gender, embarrassing. At this time, respect for female modesty and bodily privacy required male medical attendants to refrain from modes of examination that trespassed on these mores. Because of this problem, Laennec rejected the use of auscultation on the patient he was examining. What, then, to do?

Searching for an answer, he recalled both a well-known fact of acoustics, sounds grow louder when they pass through solid bodies, and an example: when one end of a solid piece of wood is scratched, the noise can be heard at the other end. Could these insights lift him over the social and physical barriers of the Hippocratic approach to auscultation and provide new evidence about his patient's illness? Spying sheets of paper nearby, he rolled them tightly into a cylinder and put one end on the region over the patient's heart and his ear on the other end. He recalled being "not a little surprised and pleased, to find that I could thereby perceive the actions of the heart in a manner much more clear and distinct than I had ever been able to do by the immediate application of the ear. From this moment I imagined that the circumstance might furnish means for enabling us to ascertain the character; not only of the actions of the heart, but of every species of sound produced by the motion of all the thoracic viscera."[7]

Laennec vigorously explored the reach and limits of his invention. Seeking to refine its makeshift character, he created instruments with different sorts of composition and construction. He found that materials of moderate density like wood, paper, and Indian cane had the best properties for hearing sounds in the body. But he also discovered that the form of his spontaneously produced initial model was the best. Thus, his chosen design was a straight wooden tube about a foot long and an inch and a half in diameter that could be separated into two parts to enhance portability. To improve his invention's sound-conducting

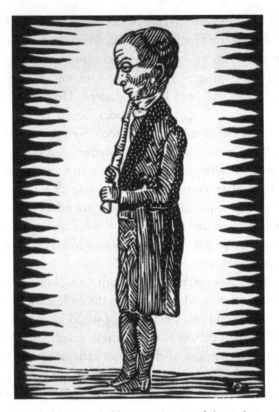

Figure 1. A caricature of Laennec holding a caricature of the stethoscope. Anonymous wood cut, 1824. Courtesy of the National Library of Medicine.

properties, the center contained a bore, which began as a quarter-inch round opening at the doctor's end and continued unchanged down its length until it neared the patient's end, where it gradually flared to almost the full diameter of the tube. The interior space thus had the configuration of a musical instrument, like a trumpet. To ensure its proper application, Laennec advised physicians to locate the hand that grasped the instrument close to the patient's body and to hold it like a pen. He called the invention "simply the cylinder, sometimes the stethoscope," the latter (from the Greek words for "chest" and "I view") being the name that became popular (Figure 1).

With the stethoscope in hand, Laennec intensely studied patients at the Necker Hospital to explore the uncharted realm of heart and lung sounds. For each disease investigated, he examined two or three patients, comparing the accuracy of diagnosis using traditional spoken and observed symptoms with that of the sounds he heard with his stetho-scope. Confirmation of the diagnosis was made by an autopsy, which demonstrated the relation between the sounds and the characteristic structural changes wrought by disease in the tissues of the body.

An example of the power of the new diagnostic technique is Laennec's discovery of a sound that confirmed the presence of the most widespread illness of his time, tuberculosis. He made the discovery while examining a woman who had a slight fever and benign cough. "On applying the cylinder below the middle of the right clavicle, while she was speaking, her voice seemed to come directly from the chest, and to reach the ear through the central canal of the instrument. This peculiar phenomenon was confined to a space about an inch square, and was not discoverable in any other part of the chest."[8] Being ignorant of its cause, Laennec examined most of the patients in the hospital at the time. He found the sign in about twenty patients, most of whom were in the advanced stages of tuberculosis. Several of those patients, however, like the woman in whom he first discovered it, had no symptoms of tuberculosis and exhibited a general robustness that appeared to rule out its presence in them. But autopsy of patients exhibiting this sign confirmed its accuracy.

Laennec declared that the sign, which he called pectoriloquism, "announced the presence of this disease [tuberculosis]... long before any other symptom leads us to suspect its existence. I may add, that it is the only sign that can be regarded as certain." People who had the basic symptoms of tuberculosis – a cough producing blood and pus, short-ness of breath, a fluctuating fever, emaciation – sometimes recovered contrary to all medical expectations. In contrast, sometimes almost all the typical symptoms of tuberculosis were absent in patients who died of it. The stethoscope, Laennec concluded, "will help us distinguish the cases which are quite beyond the resources of nature and art, from those which still leave us room to hope."[9]

Laennec worked for three years to describe the character of sounds produced in the chests of healthy and sick people. In 1819 he published his opus, which was translated into English in 1821 bearing the title *Treatise on Diseases of the Chest, and on Mediate Auscultation*. The book did far more than establish a new group of signs that physicians could use to diagnose illness. It reformulated the relationship between doctors and patients, through the use of an instrument that took the mantle of illness out of the hands of patients and placed it in the doctor's orbit. As noted, physicians had grown uneasy with and skeptical about the data patients gave them about their illnesses. Doctors recognized that some patients exaggerated the severity of their symptoms while others minimized them. Patients also might not correctly remember the sequence of events that led to or caused their symptoms. Laennec, while discussing the diagnostic significance of discharges from the body, expresses this concern: "We must never trust to the reports of patients themselves or of their attendants, as we are almost always sure of being misled by their prejudice or ignorance."[10]

Such limitations evaporated when physicians could focus on the acoustic signs of illness detected through the stethoscope. These sounds could be linked by physical principles to the anatomical lesions that produced them, while the sensations that patients experienced as symptoms had no such direct links to changes inside the body. For example, the eminent French scientist François Magendie, while experimentally investigating pathological heart sounds, found one that was produced by impediments to the passage of blood through the heart. "At least in all the post mortem examinations which I have made of patients who have exhibited this stethoscopic symptom during life," he wrote, "I have always found the pathological change now described."[11]

Advocates of the stethoscope asserted that the connection between physical principles and the acoustic signs made them more dependable than all other symptoms of chest diseases. "In truth," wrote a doctor, "the exact state of the functions of the heart and lungs cannot be ascertained except by the ear."[12] The point was reinforced in a public challenge made by a critic of the stethoscope to an advocate. The contest required both to evaluate the same patient: one with and the other without the instrument. A verdict emerged when the patient died and was autopsied. The stethoscope's champion emerged the victor.[13]

The ability of doctors to find diseases began to outstrip their ability to treat them, an imbalance that raised this question: why work to accurately diagnose an illness when effective therapy didn't exist? The answer given at that time still remains cogent. Without the knowledge that technology produced, doctors often diagnosed their patients incorrectly and treated them for the wrong diseases. Further, knowledge of the true condition from which a patient suffered, if incurable, freed doctors to halt often-aggressive treatments directed at cure and to replace them with therapies that relieved symptoms and supported and comforted the patient. The most certain guide to treatment was knowing, noted a doctor in 1836, "the situation and extent of disease."[14] At this time the stethoscope was the leading edge of such knowledge.

Despite its benefits, many doctors opposed the stethoscope. An important cause, and a factor that continues to influence the spread of a new technology in medicine, is the problem of learning its use. Several obstacles appeared, one of which was the doctor's hearing. Some practitioners insisted that to practice auscultation, "what musicians call 'a good ear' or a delicate appreciation of minute differences of sound, is an important if not essential qualification."[15] Others worried about the mental challenge of discriminating sounds that reached the ear: "The diversity of hues in a rainbow, are not harder to be remembered than the variety of sounds given out by different bodies under different circumstances. . . . Whoever aspires to be proficient with the stethoscope had better construct a gamut for himself. . . . It requires the greatest attention to avoid error. Its use can only be acquired by unremitting perseverance."[16] Laennec disputed this view. He asserted that physicians needed only to study several patients with a given illness to learn the sounds marking its presence. The consensus that emerged from this debate was that several weeks of use gave basic learning, and several months produced an educated ear.[17]

A second aspect of the learning issue that delayed the stethoscope's acceptance was an unwillingness of doctors to become students again. Even after allaying their doubts about its value, those who feared leaving the security of older learning and trying to achieve prominence with an innovation resisted the stethoscope. A doctor observed that when such colleagues spoke of having tried auscultation and found it "useless or unavailable, the just conclusion may be deduced, that the attempt was commenced in doubt, followed without interest, and relinquished in wisdom."[18]

Physicians also worried about becoming instrument users and thus associated in the public mind not only with the common trades but also with surgery. The previously noted entrance of medical studies into the university in the thirteenth century had led to a separation of surgery from medicine. United before, the textual and philosophical focus of university education led doctors to abandon and look down upon the surgical discipline, whose practice was technological and manually based. Cast out from the universities, surgeons studied mainly through apprenticeship until the mid-nineteenth century, when surgery was once again made part of medicine. This reunion was advanced by successful efforts to make the stethoscope and other technologies that would follow it commonplace elements in the work of the doctor.

Ironically, however, zealous supporters erected the greatest barrier to the acceptance of auscultation. They ignored its limitations, touted it as a universal gateway to diagnostic certainty, and demeaned the value of older diagnostic measures. By raising the expectations of those who tried the stethoscope beyond its ability to meet them, the enthusiasts sowed disillusion and fostered rejection. "Auscultation has suffered in this way from its friends," wrote a doctor.[19] The Harvard Medical School professor Oliver Wendell Holmes parodied the overconfident stethoscopist in a ballad published in 1848 called "The Stethoscope Song."[20] The song tells the tale of a doctor who went to the stethoscope's Parisian birthplace to study the instrument and returned to America entranced and, ultimately, victimized by its messages:

> There was a young man in Boston town
>   He bought him a STETHOSCOPE nice and new,
> All mounted and finished and polished down,
>   With an ivory cap and a stopper too.
>
> It happened a spider within did crawl,
>   And spun him a web of ample size,
> Wherein there chanced one day to fall
>   A couple of very imprudent flies.
>
> The first was a bottle-fly, big and blue,
>   The second was smaller, and thin and long;
> So there was a concert between the two,
>   Like an octave flute and a tavern gong.
>
> • • •
>
> There was an old lady had long been sick,
>   And what was the matter none did know;
> Her pulse was slow, though her tongue was quick;
>   To her this knowing youth must go.
>
> • • •

Now, when the stethoscope came out,
   The flies began to buzz and whiz; –
O ho! The matter is clear, no doubt;
   An *aneurism* there plainly is.

      • • •

Now, when the neighboring doctors found
   A case so rare had been descried,
They every day her ribs did pound
   In squads of twenty; so she died.

      • • •

Now use your ears, all you that can,
   But don't forget to mind your eyes;
Or you may be cheated, like this young man,
   By a couple of silly, abnormal flies.

Not only doctors put the stethoscope on trial; so did patients. Being examined with an instrument was a new experience and it made them apprehensive. Indeed, some patients, seeing a doctor holding a stethoscope approach them, thought they were about to have surgery. Even the stethoscope's basic strength – its reputation for accuracy – stirred concern. For doctors, applying this instrument would likely confirm the worst fears of patients about their illness. There was no room for hope based on error. The first stanza of the poem "To the Stethoscope" depicts its dreaded power:

Stethoscope: thou simple tube,
Clarion of the yawning tomb,
Unto me thou seem'st to be
A very trump of doom.[21]

Indeed there was then, and still is now, something enigmatic about a doctor placing a tube on one's chest, hearing sounds in the body unknown to its owner, and making pronouncements based on them.

Gradually, the patients overcame the anxieties of being examined with the stethoscope. Not only did its use become associated with exemplary practice, but doctors who failed to examine patients with it faced criticism and loss. A doctor in 1827 claimed it would be "positively suicidal" to one's professional reputation to ignore the stethoscope.[22] A practitioner unwilling to learn auscultation but concerned about public opinion was spied to assume "a look of great wisdom – apply the wrong end of the stethoscope to his ear – hold the other end about two inches from the patient's chest – and sagely remark, that he heard, very distinctly, the respiratory murmer!"[23] The sounds were in fact the wheels of a coach traveling over a newly paved road across from the patient's house.

It took about two decades after the invention of the stethoscope for auscultation to be fully accepted in medicine. Speaking of its place in Britain, the physician James Hope wrote in 1838: "Auscultation has withstood the most violent assaults that ever stormed any science, and has emerged strong and refreshed from the struggle.... The public has proclaimed its fiat; the public *will have* auscultation. The public *must* be obeyed. Auscultation is dominant in every great school and hospital in London – in every one of the English provinces and Scotland. Auscultors are in the first ranks of professional success, here and in every great town throughout Britain."[24]

The rise of the stethoscope and the triumph of auscultation is not only the story of a good idea getting its due: it is also a tale of transforming relationships. With the transfer of doctors' attention from the words spoken by patients to the sounds produced by their organs, the beginnings of modern therapeutic distancing arrived. Contemporary medicine is filled with complaints about patients not being listened to, about doctors rushing from one examining room to the other – exploring the body, writing orders for tests, and inadequately regarding the person in the patient. These doctors follow a pattern forged by the stethoscope. For the system of diagnosis that produced its birth, anchored in the anatomical lesions of disease and the quest to locate them, was scientifically exhilarating for doctors. At last they could base their opinions on facts proved true through physical principles and autopsy demonstration; facts personally gained through their own senses; facts independent of the untrustworthy memory and unpredictable will of the patient. Doctors in control of such facts felt free to independently reach medical judgments. Unfortunately, this freedom was purchased by their liberation from the subjective world of the patient.

Diagnostic technologies focus users on particular aspects of reality. The more compelling and authentic this reality seems, the greater is the user's belief that it says enough. In this way a partial perspective of a complex reality becomes an acceptable substitute for the whole. Thus, if the sound tells all, why bother with what the person thinks or feels?

However, it would not be long before the dominance of the stethoscope and its sonic evidence was challenged by a new kind of technology that swept into medicine and emerged as a rival.

2

ENIGMATIC PICTURES

How Patients and Doctors Encountered the X-Ray

Of all the photographs ever taken, probably none stirred a greater sense of awe and disbelief than a widely publicized 1895 depiction of a hand. The flesh appears as a dim translucent halo that surrounds the picture's focus – the bones. They are displayed with anatomical precision, slightly bent and poised on their joints. But the picture contains a humanizing object. The dark circle of a ring surrounds a finger and animates the hand. The picture portrays part of a living person whose exterior is stripped away. Yet how could this be? (See Figure 2.)

Stories in scientific publications and newspapers provided an answer. A phenomenon generated in a tube in a laboratory created rays that could penetrate the skin and reveal the structures beneath it, rays whose nature was unknown, and hence they were described as X. The picture announced a new technology that catapulted medicine into a visual age. The era generated remarkable images that changed the ways patients and doctors experienced illness. Pictures challenged the sonic portraits of the stethoscope as the holders of scientific truths and caused medicine to see its tasks and itself differently.

The path that led medicine to this point had begun centuries before, when it used other types of visual depiction to inform its work. During the Renaissance, with its focus on learning through examining the natural world, both artists and scientists attached importance to accurately representing and understanding human anatomy, concerns that were joined in the 1543 anatomical treatise by Andreas Vesalius, *De humani corporis fabrica*.[1] It portrayed the anatomical structures of the body with a scientific realism and beauty that left behind and outdated

14

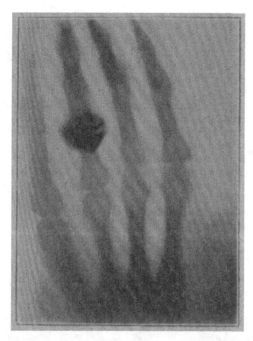

Figure 2. The first X-ray of a human being. From Wilhelm Conrad Röntgen. On a New Kind of Rays. Read before the Würzburg Physical and Medical Society in December 1895 shortly before its publication. Translated into English by Arthur Stanton. In *Nature*. 1896; 53:276. Courtesy of the National Library of Medicine.

all other efforts in this arena. The figures in the book were drawn in poses typical of Renaissance art and set against a natural background. Sections illustrating the body's muscles, nerves, blood vessels, internal organs, bones, and other tissues revealed the complexity and relationships of its structures. It was as if the interior of the human body was being seen for the first time, for most previous anatomical depictions were basically schematic representations of its structures (Figure 3).

Having started with Vesalius, drawn medical images became scientific statements. They were no longer illustrations meant to supplement written material. They were independent data held to a high standard of accuracy. In later centuries, as anatomists began to examine how normal tissues were changed by illness, and claimed that the location and appearance of this altered tissue described and captured the essence of particular diseases, the rationale to draw them accurately was established. Other anatomists and physicians would depend on those drawings to study and diagnose diseases.

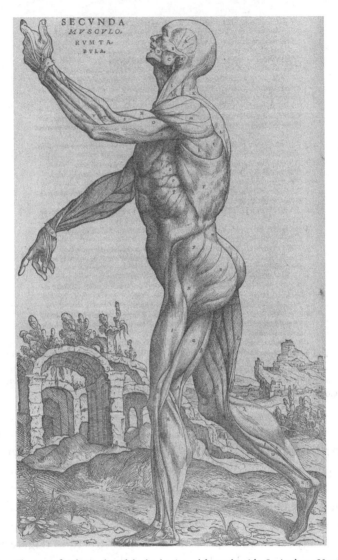

Figure 3. The superficial muscles of the body viewed from the side. In Andreas Vesalius. *De humani corporis fabrica libri septum*. Basel, 1543, 174. Courtesy of the National Library of Medicine.

In the seventeenth century, the invention of the microscope brought doctors into another visual world. It revealed biological structures hidden from the naked eye. Their architecture displayed a stunning array of intricate patterns and complexities. In one of the earliest works on the subject, *Micrographia*, written in 1665, Robert Hooke drew a section

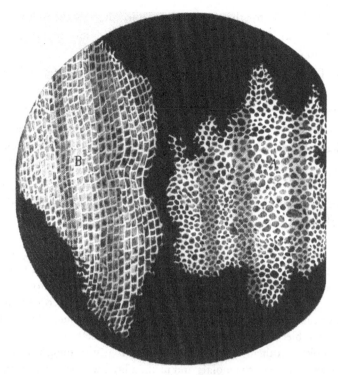

Figure 4. "Cells" of cork seen through a microscope. In Robert Hooke. *Micrographia; or, Some Physiological Descriptions of Minute Bodies Made by Magnifying Glasses*. London: Jo. Marten and Ja. Allestry, 1665. Courtesy of the National Library of Medicine.

of cork.[2] He had in fact discovered a basic building block of life – the cell – and he depicted it but without grasping its biological significance (Figure 4).

Others soon followed Hooke in making discoveries about this new world. One of the first medical advances made with the microscope was finding the cause of the common skin disorder scabies (popularly called "the itch"). In 1687 the Italian doctor Giovanni Bonomo, after he saw children with the disorder use a pin to pull tiny water-filled sacs from their skin, determined to look at the material with the microscope: "I quickly found an *itchy* person, and asking him where he felt the greatest and most acute *itching*...I took out a very small *globule*, scarcely discernible. Observing this with a microscope, I found it to be a living creature, in shape, resembling a tortoise, of whitish colour, a little dark upon the back, with some thin and long hairs, of nimble motion, with six feet, a sharp head, two little horns at the end of the snout." The reason for the extreme contagiousness of the itch was now clear to Bonomo. The organisms jumped from person to person, "their motion being wonderfully swift."[3]

As did scientists investigating anatomy visible to the naked eye, microscopists increasingly used the art of drawing to show the results of their work. One of them was Antoni van Leeuwenhoek, a Dutch lens maker who perfected monocular microscopes and investigated many biological objects with them. In letters written to the Royal Society of London in the mid-1670s, he described tiny living organisms floating in water, probably the first observation of bacteria. In the early 1680s, however, he found the tiny creatures living in the human body. He writes about this in a letter dated September 17, 1683:

I am in the habit of rubbing my teeth in the morning, and then swill out my mouth with water; and often after eating, to clean my back teeth with a toothpick, as well as rubbing them hard with a cloth, wherefore my teeth back and front remain as clean and white that only a few people of my age (fifty-one) can compare with me. Also when I rub my gums with hard salt, they will not bleed. Yet all this does not make my teeth so clean but that I can see, looking at them with a hollow mirror, that something will stick and grow between some of the molars and teeth, a little white matter, as thick as batter. Observing it I judged that although I could not see anything moving in it there were yet living animalcules in it. I then mixed it several times with pure rain-water, in which there were no animalcules, and also with saliva that I took from my mouth after eliminating the air bubbles lest these should stir the spittle. I then again and again saw that there were many small living animalcules in the said matter, which moved very prettily.[4]

Accompanying the letter are drawings, the first ones of bacteria, which depict them as various-sized creatures having round and oblong shapes.

In the 1830s an alternative to this form of illustration emerged with the invention of photography. It rapidly became a medium used by artists as an alternative to drawing and painting, and by the 1850s it had found a place in medicine. Doctors photographed patients to show typical presentations of illness, and they took pictures of themselves to describe who they were, what they did, and where they worked.[5] Gradually, scientists also saw important applications for photography in studying disease, particularly the German investigator Robert Koch. In 1880 he initiated a series of experiments to test the long-standing idea that human disease was caused by bacteria. He labored for two years in his laboratory and in 1882 announced a discovery that changed the course of medicine. He had unmasked the source of tuberculosis, the main illness and cause of death in his time. The culprit was a minute organism shaped like a rod, which he named the tubercle bacillus. To establish the validity of his discovery, and conclusively demonstrate the role of bacteria as causes of disease, Koch employed a complicated series of proofs, central to which was photography.

A great problem of using the microscope at that time was that different observers of a particular object, who used different microscopes and viewed phenomena under different conditions, reached diverse and often contradictory conclusions when viewing the same specimens. The inability of microscopists in distant laboratories to communicate about their findings compounded the problem. Koch was critical of drawing objects to preserve microscopical findings. The drawings seemed always to present objects more sharply and structured than they appeared to the observer, and they were susceptible to manipulations, conscious or unconscious, that reflected the views of their makers.

Photography entered as rescuer. Koch believed that in some instances a photograph was superior to the direct observation of the specimen itself. A photograph created an image of the specimen at the precise level of magnification and sharpness desired. It produced a fixed depiction of the object that could be shared with other observers in the same and distant laboratories. They could discuss the image together and reach a consensus on what was there.[6]

By the 1880s photography had become a fixed part of other professional cultures. It was used by police in their crime-fighting efforts, by the military in reconnaissance, by artists to create images of people and landscapes, by anthropologists to document their cultural studies, by journalists and newspapers to report on events of the day, and so forth. The complexity of taking pictures using large cameras and cumbersome glass-plate negatives essentially restricted its use to professional purposes. In 1888 an inexpensive and easy-to-use camera, the Kodak, was invented by George Eastman. Instead of glass plates, it employed a celluloid strip wound on a spool as film. It was placed in a small and readily portable wooden box with a fixed lens, which put objects eight or more feet from it in sharp focus. Customers were offered the option of returning the camera to Eastman to develop and print the film ("You press the button, we do the rest" was the company slogan). The invention inaugurated the age of popular photography.[7]

It was into this environment that the X-ray picture of the hand entered. In October 1895 its maker, Wilhelm Röntgen, professor of physics and director of the physics institute at the University of Würzburg, became interested in the ongoing scientific investigations of the phenomenon of cathode rays. These were produced when electric currents were discharged in tubes from which the air had been partially removed by a vacuum pump and inside of which were placed a positive and a negative electrode. To study the properties of these cathode rays outside of the tube (called a Crookes tube), experimenters inserted a thin aluminum window that permitted the rays to disperse into the outside air. It was found, however, that the rays migrated only a few centimeters beyond the tube.

Röntgen repeated these experiments and apparently confirmed this short-range migration by the effects the rays produced on a cardboard screen painted with a fluorescing chemical. He then wondered whether a Crookes tube without the thin window might also emit cathode rays, detectable on the cardboard screen but missed by previous investigators because of luminescence produced within the tube itself. In the late afternoon of November 8, 1895, Röntgen tested this idea. He covered a Crookes tube with black cardboard, darkened the room, and discharged the tube with electric current to check the effectiveness of the cover. It emitted no light. He was about to stop the current and set up the fluorescing screen for his experiment when he noted light coming from a nearby bench. Puzzled, he stopped and again sent a series of currents through the tube. Once more, light appeared, as faint green clouds flickering in consonance with the discharges of current. He lit a match and found that the light source was his fluorescent screen lying on the bench about a yard away. He repeated the experiment, placing the screen at increasing distances from the tube. The screen continued to flicker. He pondered the results. Cathode rays had never been reported to migrate that far. What, then, could account for his observations? He dwelt on the question for hours in the laboratory and was finally induced by his wife to come to dinner.[8]

Over several weeks, Röntgen repeated his experiment and probed the properties of the mysterious emanation, including its transit through solid objects. He found that it traveled through paper. "I observed that the fluorescent screen still glowed brightly behind a bound book of about 1000 pages." The emanations, which he decided to call X-rays, because he did not know their composition, passed also through sheets of tinfoil and rubber, and thick blocks of wood, glass, and aluminum. But they failed to penetrate other objects such as lead. He produced also what he called shadow pictures, by placing material between the X-ray apparatus and photographic plates, which he found were sensitive to the rays. This was an important discovery: "One is able to make a permanent record of many phenomena whereby deceptions are more easily avoided; and as a control I have, wherever possible, recorded every relatively important observation that I saw on the fluorescent screen by means of photography," wrote Röntgen.[9]

He took shadow pictures of objects such as a compass encased in metal (Figure 5), weights resting in a wooden box, a wire wound around a wooden spool, a piece of metal whose internal flaws were revealed, and the bones of the hand. He thought of bones as a possible subject when, while holding a piece of lead to test the ray's effect on it, he saw the bony outline of his own thumb and finger on the fluorescent screen. This led him to ask his wife to participate in an experiment: to place her hand on a cassette containing a photographic plate for fifteen minutes while directing X-rays at it. Wrote Röntgen's biographer, Otto Glasser: "When he showed the picture to her, she could hardly believe the bony hand was her own and shuddered at the thought that she was seeing her own skeleton. To Frau Roentgen, as to many others later, this experience gave a vague premonition of death."[10]

On December 28, 1895, Röntgen presented to the secretary of the Würzburg Physical-Medical Society his manuscript "On a New Kind of Rays, A Preliminary Communication" for the society's journal. Its significance prompted the secretary to place it in the issue that was about to come out. To hasten disclosure, Röntgen sent reprints of his paper to colleagues on January 1, 1896, along with some of the photographs taken with X-rays. The discovery was now revealed.

The public immediately recognized the discovery's implications for the treatment of illness. Early newspaper stories reported on the possible use of X-rays to detect fractures without requiring the painful manual

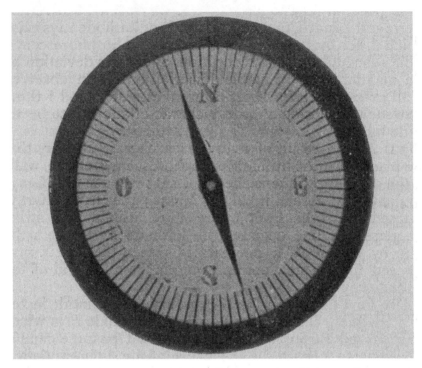

Figure 5. Röntgen's X-ray through metal (1895). A simple picture demonstrates the X-ray's extraordinary power to a late-nineteenth-century scientific and public audience: an ability to see the card and needle of a compass totally enclosed in a metal case. From Wilhelm Conrad Röntgen. On a New Kind of Rays. Read before the Würzburg Physical and Medical Society in December 1895 shortly before its publication. Translated into English by Arthur Stanton. In *Nature*. 1896; 53:276. Courtesy of the National Library of Medicine.

examination of the break in the bone to determine their severity and extent. They pragmatically speculated about detecting the location of objects such as bullets in the body without needing painful manual probing for them. Some people also were anxious over the possibility of having their privacy violated. This concern led to X-ray-proof under-garments being offered for sale in London and to a legislative proposal in New Jersey forbidding the use of X-ray-equipped opera glasses in the-aters. Businesses seized on the public's interest in the discovery. In New York, Bloomingdale Brothers department store opened an exhibition to demonstrate X-rays.[11] X-ray apparatuses also were displayed in shop windows as curiosities. X-ray photographs of ordinary objects such as keys in purses were sold. Couples holding hands were photographed with X-rays and their bony portraits given to family members.[12]

A month after the announcement of the discovery, the newspaper publisher William Randolph Hearst telegraphed Thomas Alva Edison: "Will you as an especial favor to the journal undertake to make a cathodograph of human brain. Kindly telegraph answer at our expense." Edison accepted the invitation and created great popular expectation and excitement that he would photograph "the living brain."[13] Yet the thickness of the skull bones presented a barrier he could not overcome, no matter how he tried to augment Röntgen's technology. After two months, his effort ended in failure.

In early 1896, the Mountain Electric Company in Colorado invited the public in to have free X-rays. It was "besieged by persons who were certain that their physicians were wrong, and wanted X-ray photographs to prove it." The company changed its policy and gave X-rays only to individuals who came with their doctors.[14]

The reaction of physicians and scientists to Röntgen's discovery was equally enthusiastic. Speaking before the Medical Society of the County of New York several months after Röntgen's announcement, Dr. William J. Martin said: "Physicians, from time immemorial have ever had a keen desire to explore the interior of the animal body. Hence arose dissection, and later on vivisection, and still later on the revelations of the microscope. But none of these methods fully satisfy the wish to know what is actually taking place within the animal organism during life.... No wonder then that the X-ray with its marvelous revelations of the hitherto unseen has excited a universal interest."[15]

A professor at the University of Pennsylvania, Henry Cattell, wrote in March 1896: "It is even now questionable whether a surgeon would be morally justified in performing a certain class of operations without first having seen pictured by these rays the field of his work – a map, as it were, of the unknown country he is to explore." As the year progressed, X-rays were used to diagnose a broad range of ailments. In the span of a month, doctors at McGill University in Montreal examined a child with a bullet in the brain, a man with a broken hip, a patient in whose lung a drainage tube had been lost, a patient with a possible skull fracture who had been gored by a bull several years earlier, one with a cavity in the lungs, and another with symptoms of kidney stones. In addition to such patients who presented with difficult diagnostic problems, the doctors X-rayed a large number of patients for simple fractures.[16]

But the embrace of the X-ray by the public and professional communities also had a dark side, which took decades to fully grasp. In the first year of the X-ray's use, reports emerged of damage to the health of those working with it. The demonstrator of X-rays in the Bloomingdale Brothers department store, for example, suffered significant burns to the skin and hair, as well as memory loss from continued exposure to them. Scientists and physicians using X-rays reported similar experiences. While those working with the rays were moved by the reports to take at least minimal precautions, the public getting X-rayed was reassured about safety: "No harmful effects have been received in any way by the patients, more than 250 in number, whom I have examined by the X-rays at this hospital, and there need not be the slightest anxiety on the part of the patient if the examinations are made by someone who has had experience and has suitable apparatus," wrote Boston City Hospital X-ray pioneer Francis Williams in 1897.[17]

Swept up by the extraordinary insights into the interior of the body given by X-rays and lulled by their apparent harmlessness when an individual received them in small doses, the medical world and public began to fully explore and appreciate their harmful side only when the atomic bomb and the dawn of the nuclear age at the end of the Second World War raised awareness of the dangers of radiation. But even with this heightened sensitivity, the rays continued to be treated casually by the public. Nothing typified this attitude more than the X-ray devices found in American and British shoe stores starting in the mid-1920s that allowed customers to see the bones and soft tissues of their feet and the fit of the shoes they were trying. An American doctor who invented one of those machines, Jacob Lowe, declared in 1927: "With this apparatus in his shop, a shoe merchant can positively assure his customers that they never need wear ill-fitting boots and shoes; that parents can visually assure themselves as to whether they are buying shoes for their boys and girls which will not injure and deform the sensitive bone joints." The X-ray fitting of shoes reached its zenith in the early 1950s in the United States, when about ten thousand machines were in use. Only by the decade's end were they discredited, when many states banned their use.[18] This was well after the danger of radiation and the need to limit X-ray exposure had been established.

When the risks associated with a valued benefit are not immediately sensed and are far off, a rationale exists for throwing caution to the wind, and this the public did with regard to the X-ray. The cellular damage the rays could produce was not felt by people, and the development of illness from them could take decades to occur. The response of the public was aided by doctors, who had developed a reliance on the X-ray for diagnosis as a result of both a strong belief in the evidence it gave and a loss of skills and confidence in alternatives to it, such as the physical examination.

This was illustrated in the mid-1930s when the chief of radiology at the Peter Bent Brigham Hospital in Boston had a display case containing a stethoscope built and installed in the X-ray viewing room. Two labels were affixed to the case. One read, "Valuable specimen – Please Do Not Touch." The other said: "Rare and unusually well preserved fragments of an instrument known as the 'stethescope' [sic] (binaural type circa 1918) formerly in common use in the diagnosis of pulmonary and cardiac disease. The contraption was developed by Laennec early in the 19th century and was actually in general use until the Röntgen era."[19]

In 1945 the Royal Society of Medicine in London sponsored a debate on the merits of the stethoscope versus X-rays. The consensus of participants was that the stethoscope's value had seriously declined, and they asked, theoretically, why physicians should concern themselves with "vague mysterious sounds, when something quite definite could be seen on the X-ray film?"[20] Gradually, doctors viewed X-ray examinations as superior to all other forms of medical analysis. By 1961 physicians asserted that "to a phenomenal degree X-rays have been used to amplify older methods of physical examination as well as to supercede them with unique diagnostic procedures entirely dependent on the X-ray principle."[21]

In our own time, this thinking continues. Wrote a doctor in 2002:

It is a common scene at teaching hospitals today: young doctors ignoring physical examination to the chagrin of their supervisors. At one time, keen observation and the judicious laying on of hands were virtually the only diagnostic tools a doctor had. Now, they seem almost obsolete. Technology like ultra fast CAT scans and nuclear imaging studies rule the day, permitting diagnosis at a distance. Some doctors don't even carry a stethoscope anymore. If postmodernism teaches that there are many truths, or perhaps no truth, postmodern medicine teaches the opposite: that objective truth will explain a patient's symptoms, if we look for it with the right tools.[22]

That is the problem: a belief that objective medical findings can fully answer the question of what is wrong with patients. However, this idea did not arise in contemporary times. Its origin in medicine goes back to the turn of the nineteenth century, to events that produced the dominance of a technology that modern doctors are ready to discard – the stethoscope.

Recall that Laennec and the physicians who elevated stethoscopic findings over evidence gained from the stories patients told rejected narrative evidence because it was subjective – personally derived, verbal, and unverifiable. Who knew whether patients truly felt the symptoms they reported, or when they really started, or how troubling they really were? The illness narratives given by patients existed in memory, which could be flawed; they were stated in words, which could be wrongly chosen; and they were influenced by personal motives, which could not be fathomed by medical observers.

Enter the stethoscope. No need to probe the depth of human experience nor worry about the accuracy with which it was described. The technology permitted doctors to independently access pathology in the body through the act of placing a simple tool on it. The body revealed what was wrong by the sounds it made. No concern here about forgetfulness, fabrication, or motives. Sounds, pure and physical, reached the ears of doctors, who alone analyzed their significance – isolated from the personality and will of patients, in tune only with their own physiological self.

The stethoscope liberated doctors from patients and, by doing so, paradoxically enabled doctors to think they helped them better. This was the logic of the physical examination. Listening to the body seemed to get one further diagnostically than did listening to the patient.

The X-ray challenged the hegemony of the stethoscope by introducing a new form of realism – the photograph. Photography was more than fifty years old when X-rays were discovered. By that time, photographs had acquired a reputation as objective representations of things as they were. In artistic circles, they were compared with paintings and thought to be aesthetically inferior. Artists with brush, paint, and canvas were free to introduce creative, subjective elements into their work. Anything that their mind and experience suggested was interesting could be put on the canvas in ways of their choosing. Mind and medium created intensely subjective visual statements. Not so with photography. The lens of the camera projected onto photographic plates or film what really was there. The subjective decision made in producing a photograph was where to point the lens – after that, automation took over. The resulting picture was therefore an objective and unbiased statement of reality.

At the time the X-ray was invented, it not only carried the prevailing ideology about the photograph's nature. It also was born in a scientific laboratory, described by a prominent investigator, and revealed in a journal of physics. With such a heritage, the X-ray entered medicine with significant standing as an objective depiction of illness. So if ordinary photographs did not lie, this surely was also true of X-rays. The quotations from the medical literature cited previously bear out the tenacity of this perspective in the more than one hundred years of their clinical use. But there are troubling issues to confront. Are X-rays really objective? Is their evidence sufficient to understand illness? The answer to each question is no, and here is why.

One of the best statements on the meaning of objectivity in the modern era was made in 1900 in a book written by the mathematician Karl Pearson, *The Grammar of Science*.[23] Pearson defines the "scientific frame of mind" as the ability of a person to eliminate the self from judgments and thus make objective statements about the world. It was on this ground that the findings of the stethoscope were challenged by the proponents of X-rays. Auscultation with the stethoscope was based on what the doctor heard through it. Yet who but the auscultors could know what they really heard, and how did anyone know whether that represented accurately the sounds generated by the body? How could the auscultors remove the self from their description of body sounds when hearing and transcribing them into words was wholly dependent on this self? Ironically, the very criticism on which auscultors based their disregard of the narrative account of illness by the patient – that it was tainted by the subjectivity of transcribing sensations into words – now was turned back on them.

The power of the photograph was its seeming ability to transcend these limitations by objectively capturing reality. The art critic John Berger wrote of this: "Unlike any other visual image, a photograph is not a rendering, an imitation or an interpretation of its subject, but actually a trace of it. No painting or drawing, however naturalistic, belongs to its subject in the way that a photograph does."[24] This was the view of the X-ray held by its medical pioneers and early subjects, and it continues to prevail today. The authenticity of the X-ray is based on doctors' and patients' belief in a connection to reality that surpasses other forms of medical evidence.

The flaw in this thinking is demonstrated by ideas that were first expressed in the nineteenth century but that were not evaluated comprehensively until the twentieth century. Their focus is the circumstances in medical evaluations that produce variations and errors in judgment. Some nineteenth-century physicians recognized that differences in the construction of their technologies and in the perceptions of observers viewing the same object could produce mistakes and dissension, a phenomenon noted in our earlier discussion of the microscope. Studies of this issue were undertaken in the twentieth century, one of the most fascinating and influential of which involved the X-ray.

In 1947 an investigation was made of the accuracy of the small X-ray films used during the Second World War to speed up the mass screening of military recruits. Participants, however, were stunned by a revelation that appeared as a side effect of the study. To evaluate the X-rays, a group of radiologists was asked to read the same X-rays to be sure that no single individual's beliefs would distort the findings. They found that they differed in interpretations of the films about a third of the time and, more startling, with themselves on a second reading of the films about a fifth of the time.[25] With dismay about the outcome, a panel of three internationally distinguished radiologists was appointed to repeat the experiment. The result was the same.[26]

Such studies have been done on virtually all major diagnostic techniques, and a similar variance in human judgments has been displayed. We now know that the precision of diagnostic technologies rests on three criteria: their intrinsic accuracy, the constancy of the phenomena they measure, and the observer's ability to interpret and record the data.[27] However, these insights receive inadequate attention in medicine and are generally unknown to patients. Patients' need to believe in the reliability of technology is strong.

The views of Berger about the photograph and of physicians and patients about the X-ray do not take account of the three elements determining the precision of technologies. Changes in the composition of film, in the development process, in the placement of the X-ray camera and subject, in the anatomy and physiology of the subjects themselves, and in the views and biases of the person taking the picture influence the outcome. There is no more basic precision in the process of creating an X-ray than there is in its interpretation. A photograph or X-ray may look real but in essential ways fail to capture an object or person. We cannot escape our subjectivity. It is built into our inventions and our interpretations of them. All medical evaluations blend opinions and factual realities.

There are different kinds of truths in medicine. The illness narrative connects doctors with what, over time, the patient believes happened and why. It is the truth of personal meaning. The doctor's impressions of illness gained by sensory exploration of the body through physical examination can reveal pathologies undetected by other means and, through manual contact – a laying on of hands – can forge a link with the patient that encourages healing. This is the truth of physical connection. The technological examination is more impersonal, but the trappings and realities of the high science attached to it are reassuring to patients and valuable in diagnosis. This is the truth of scientific analysis. The context of each kind of examination and the results they produce are different. They are most valuable when taken together and most imperfect when used alone. Why, then, does it so often happen that one kind of examination is elevated over and destructive of another? What prevents medicine from achieving in succeeding generations a cumulative vision of illness, with older techniques complementing newer ones? Why is there so little effort to find ways to link the undiminished value of older technologies with the newly established benefits of new ones? Is this what is best for patients?

To establish their merits, the advocates of new technologies find it convenient, even essential, to diminish the value of the technology they wish to replace. Advocates of the stethoscope attacked the value of the patient's story. Adherents of the X-ray demeaned the salience of the stethoscope and the doctor's senses. It has become the norm in the battle for the succession of technologies in medicine to have winners and losers. Also a significant factor in this story is a vision held for centuries by doctors: of medicine becoming a science and thus eliminating subjective elements when they seem to be replaceable with objective ones. Scientific truth had been placed in opposition to other medical truths.

Overcoming such obstacles and mind-sets to achieve a cumulative and synthetic vision of care that integrates the technologies and truths of medicine is a continuing challenge, but one that it is essential to meet and transcend. It is an issue we will engage as our analysis of technology continues.

3

LIFESAVING BUT UNAFFORDABLE
The Improbable Journey of the Artificial Kidney

To a room in a Seattle medical center in the early 1960s came seven people to discuss the fate of patients. They were not a medical team, but women and men from diverse occupations brought together to select recipients for a new lifesaving technology – kidney dialysis. It was not their job to judge who among the many claimants was most medically able to benefit from the technology. That issue had been addressed by a panel of medical experts who had assembled a pool of clinically acceptable candidates for the laypeople to consider. Their task was to introduce a community perspective into the rationing decision, necessitated by the limits caused by the great expense of dialysis. In effect, the citizens had to apply their values to the question of who in their community should be saved from dying. Even now – almost a half century after this event and in a time filled with intense public debate about the rights and wrongs of using technologies for purposes such as determining a person's genetic destiny and prolonging the lives of deeply comatose patients – the image of ordinary people in Seattle making extraordinary choices produces both awe and unease.

Ironically, an era of conflict, the Second World War, spawned the creation of an effective artificial kidney and led to the unusual circumstance of peacetime rationing. The artificial kidney was the catalyst that forced American society to grapple with the new dilemma of how patients who needed high-technology care could afford access to it.

At the start of the Second World War, Willem Kolff, who grew up in a doctor's family and in early life aspired to be a zoo director, had just graduated from medical school and assumed a post as a volunteer assistant doctor in a medical clinic at the University of Groningen in the Netherlands.[1] His initial responsibility was for patients in four of its beds, one of whom was a young man dying from kidney failure. His disease had made him blind, and he suffered from constant bouts of nausea and vomiting. Writes Kolff:

His old mother was the wife of a poor farmer, her back bent by hard work, dressed in her traditional Sunday black dress, but with a very pretty white lace cap. I had to tell her that her only son was going to die, and I felt very helpless. Gradually, the idea grew in me that if we could only remove 20 g[rams] of urea and other retention products per day we might relieve this man's nausea, and that if we did this from day to day life might still be possible. This was in 1938, and soon afterwards I met Doctor R. Brinkman, Professor of Biochemistry, who showed me the wonders of cellophane.[2]

The source of this wonderment was the ability of cellophane to separate the body's own vital cellular components from waste products of body metabolism that a decline in kidney function caused to accumulate in the blood. The concept of separating materials in a liquid by passing it through a membrane, which kept larger molecules on one side and allowed smaller ones to diffuse through its pores to a liquid in the other side, was first described by the chemist Thomas Graham in an 1854 paper titled "Osmotic Force." Graham experimented with parchment and pig bladder as membranes and used the word *dialysis* to describe the transit of particles through a membrane from one fluid to another.[3] Other scientists soon expanded Graham's membrane research, particularly developing new materials and means to control the diffusion rate of fluids being dialyzed, and in the twentieth century this work was applied to medicine.[4]

Early agents of this effort were a trio of American investigators – Abel, Rountree, and Turner – who in 1913 succeeded in extracting waste substances from the blood of living animals. They used a membrane made of collodion shaped into tubes and surrounded by a salt solution. The tubes and fluid were encased in glass and connected around a cylinder. A material called hirudin, which Abel produced by crushing the heads of leeches, was introduced to prevent the coagulation of the blood as it flowed into the machine and was returned to the body. They called this device an artificial kidney. A number of investigators now began to probe the biological problems of dialyzing blood and the technological challenges of bringing this knowledge to the treatment of patients.[5]

A key figure was the German doctor George Haas, who in 1914 began to study dialysis in animals at the University of Giessen in Germany. His scientific work was interrupted in 1915 when he was drafted into the army. The death from kidney failure of many soldiers he saw in field hospitals stirred him at the war's end to develop a workable artificial kidney and achieve a result he thought akin to rinsing the blood. In 1924 he performed the first dialysis of a human being, treating two patients having kidney failure with his machine, the second and longest for thirty minutes. The main problem he faced was the inadequacy of the blood anticoagulant hirudin. Its properties placed limits on the treatment time for dialysis, and it could cause allergic reactions in patients. By 1927 he had found an answer in the recently discovered drug heparin, which he used for the first time in the dialysis of a patient. But by 1928, disheartened by the scant notice and little support given to his work, he relinquished his efforts.

While doing his studies, Haas had consulted with another German doctor, Heinrich Necheles. As did Haas, Necheles had seen the devastating effects of kidney failure on soldiers and was impelled to seek ways to cleanse the blood of debilitating wastes retained when kidneys failed. His main contribution, made through work on animals, was the development of an artificial kidney that maximized the surface area over which the blood to be dialyzed flowed and minimized the space in which this flow occurred by compressing it between screens. This was critical because the waste products the kidney machine was designed to remove required them to flow close to the dialyzing membrane to pass through it. Necheles's ideas on increasing the power of dialysis machines by affecting the flow of blood through them would be central in creating successful machines in the future.

Despite the advances made in the 1920s, the membrane that separated body waste from blood cells remained a problem. Many materials had been tested, and collodion seemed the best. But the collodion membrane tubes through which flowed the blood to be dialyzed had to be molded by the investigators themselves, and this handmade feature caused variance in the thickness of their walls – a crucial disparity in a process dependent on a certain rate of diffusion through the wall of the tubes. Into this picture in the mid-1930s came William Thalhimer, a student of Abel who became interested in the artificial kidney and focused on the membrane issue. He began experiments using cellulose acetate or cellophane membrane tubing, a product in use at the time as a casing for sausages. It had the advantage of being a manufactured material, uniform in thickness, inexpensive, strong, and readily obtainable in any quantity desired. While scientists since the mid-1920s had been investigating the properties of cellophane for use as a membrane in biological experiments, Thalhimer established its reliability for kidney dialysis.[6]

But Thalhimer was not alone in his clinical interest in cellophane tubing. Another investigator in the field of dialysis also attracted to this substance was Robert Brinkman, a professor of medical biochemistry at the University of Groningen. He was the senior professor whom the young physician Willem Kolff consulted in 1938 after his life-changing experience with the youthful patient he could not help, and he introduced Kolff to the potential of cellophane. Brinkman became a collaborator, mentor, and supporter of Kolff as he began the studies that established the artificial kidney as a major technology in medicine.[7]

Kolff not only spoke with Brinkman but also absorbed the literature of the field, reading the papers of Abel's group, Haas, Thalhimer, Necheles, and others. He concluded from his review that dialysis efforts of the past had failed for want of three essential and linked ingredients: a reliable anticoagulant, an appropriate dialyzing membrane, and a machine with adequate dialyzing power. "Since I had both heparin and cellophane," Kolff wrote, "all that remained to do was to build a dialyzer of sufficient capacity to make the application clinically worthwhile."[8]

Kolff set to work, with the help of Brinkman, to develop an artificial kidney with enhanced dialyzing capacity. The two devised an experiment to learn how much power they needed to build into the machine, in which they added the waste product urea to blood contained in a cellophane tube and placed it on a board, immersed in a solution of salt. The board itself was rocked by a motor, agitating both the blood and the salt water in an effort to enhance the diffusion of urea. After fifteen minutes all the urea left the blood and passed into the salt solution. From this work, the rate at which blood should move into the cellophane tubing and the dimensions of the tubing needed to remove a given amount of urea per minute could be calculated. A second construction requirement for the dialyzer also discerned was that blood must be able to flow into and out of it easily.

With the data from such experiments, Kolff both built and had made several artificial kidneys. But he suffered the double misfortune of having to pay for their construction himself and finding them afterward to be inadequate for clinical use. It was then that war began. On May 10, 1940, Germany invaded the Netherlands. Kolff, in another part of the country at this time, was cut off from returning to his house in Groningen. So to help the war effort, he remained where he was, went to a local hospital, and offered to create a blood bank for it; he did this in four days and then established one in Groningen on his return. This experience had the favorable side effect of giving him "confidence in handling blood outside the body, and this is exactly what one does with an artificial kidney."[9]

In 1941 Kolff left Groningen for a post in the city of Kampen as the first internist in its ninety-bed hospital. The hospital's board of governors complied with Kolff's request for a modern laboratory staffed by several technicians on duty around the clock to perform chemical analyses for patient care. The availability of such data at any time of the day or night later proved important in Kolff's efforts to develop an effective artificial kidney. So, too, did his authority as head of his own department and a private practice that generated income to support his research.

He now determined to press ahead with his life mission of creating a machine to effectively treat kidney failure. He collaborated with H. Th. J. Berk, director of the largest industry in town, the Kampen Enamel Works, who persuaded Kolff to change the orientation of the drum around which the dialyzing cellophane tubing membrane would be wound from a vertical to a horizontal direction. In this model, blood would sink in the tubing to the lowest point of the drum, and as it rotated, the blood would be forced through the action of gravity to continually seek this low point and thus run through the cellophane tubing from end to end. The drum itself was immersed in a liquid into which the body wastes would diffuse. This arrangement also caused both the blood to be dialyzed and the liquid into which the waste products would flow to remain in constant motion, a factor Kolff had recognized from earlier experiments as essential for effective dialysis.

The stage was set for a clinical test, which occurred on March 17, 1943. Kolff's first patient was a twenty-nine-year-old woman in a dire condition from failing kidneys and an accompanying extremely high blood pressure and failing vision. To Kolff and her doctors, there seemed nothing to lose in giving over her care to an untested therapy, which might at least improve her condition in the short term. Kolff started by removing increasingly large amounts of the patient's blood over a five-day period, passing it through the artificial kidney and then injecting it back into her. This was done to determine whether the dialysis process produced serious adverse reactions. Kolff's assistant at this time, Jakob van Noordwijk (who later became his biographer), describes the unfolding drama after the first such quotient of blood drawn and collected from the patient was placed in a glass tube containing heparin to prevent clotting and put into the machine. It begins with a request to him from Kolff to initiate dialysis:

"Switch it on, will you." I switched on the motor, and the drum started to rotate. A soft humming filled the room and mingled with the rustling of water in the tank, that was set in motion by the rotating drum. The colourless fluid in the cellophane tube around the drum became dark red at the end where the blood flowed into it. The blood kept on sinking to the lowest part of the cellophane tube and so that red colour moved on through all the windings of the cellophane tube until the whole outside of the drum looked red. As the blood moved through the cellophane tube the colour became somewhat lighter. The blood left the cellophane tube via a rubber tube through the hollow axle of the drum and then it was returned to the beginning so that it had to follow its way through the cellophane tube again.

After some 20 minutes Dr. Kolff decided to stop. The blood was collected again in the glass tube and siphoned back into the patient's vein. At his sign I switched off the motor. The rustling of the water ended; for some moments some water dripped from the drum back into the tank – the rest was silence.[10]

Determining, after a five-day trial, that the dialyzed blood did not harm the patient when it was returned to her body, Kolff began continuous dialysis, with blood from the patient entering the machine and returning directly from it to her. While the patient gained benefits from the dialysis, the machine could not save her life.

From March 1943 through July 1944, Kolff treated fifteen patients with the artificial kidney. Only one survived, a result that Kolff did not believe was produced by his therapy. However, like the first patient, a number experienced relief from their symptoms. The fifth patient became wakeful, spoke to his family with renewed clarity, and made a will. Another patient, who had been brought to Kolff extremely ill, got well enough to read a newspaper. "Most striking," wrote Kolff, "and this we were very much aware of – was the improvement in the sensorum of our patients."[11]

There were other clinical benefits, too. Vomiting diminished in many of the cases and urinary output improved. From the viewpoint of the patients' physiological status, dialysis markedly decreased the blood content of the major waste products caused by kidney failure, such as urea. It also rebalanced the proportions of important blood chemicals such as salt, chlorine, and potassium. These biochemical and clinical improvements, the absence of alternative measures to apply in kidney failure, and the hope that a therapy giving more time in life might also produce a cure account for the persistence of referring doctors, willing patients, and their families to seek this therapy and for Kolff to agree to give it.

Conditions in the Netherlands in the last year of the war made artificial kidney treatment impossible. But Kolff resumed it several months after it ended and had a breakthrough with his seventeenth patient, whom he treated on September 11, 1945. The patient was a sixty-seven-year-old woman who was unconscious and had stopped passing urine from a combination of gall bladder and kidney disorders. She improved dramatically during an eleven and a half hour period on the kidney machine and then began to speak. "The first understandable words she spoke that I remember," recalled Kolff, "were that she was going to divorce her husband, which indeed in time she did."[12]

Kolff's work had to overcome not only the hurdles of a journey into the scientific unknown but also the trials of a wartime environment, which created shortages and tested courage. Shortages of rubber and glass tubing, essential in connecting patient and machine, and leaks in the cellophane tubing (once caused by dropping a scissors on the kidney machine) were typical of the technical dilemmas Kolff faced. Equally difficult were Nazi threats and intimidation, which Kolff resisted. He went underground for a short time after refusing to sign a declaration of allegiance to Germany, and he was instrumental in keeping from

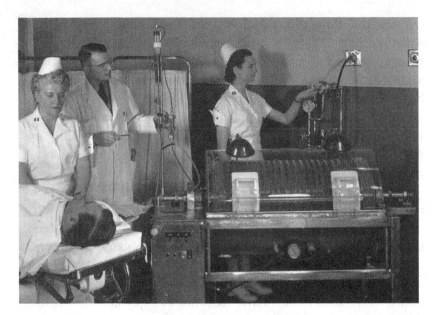

Figure 6. Dialysis of a patient with a Kolff-Brigham artificial kidney at the Walter Reed Army Medical Center in Washington, D.C. (ca. 1951–1952). Photograph by William Warrell. Courtesy of Otis Historical Archive, National Museum of Health and Medicine, Armed Forces Institute of Pathology, Washington, D.C.

In 1947 Willem Kolff visited the Harvard-affiliated Peter Bent Brigham Hospital in Boston and faced a quandary. He no longer had kidney machines in his possession but wished to make his invention available there. "All I could do," he wrote, "was to present blueprints to Dr. Carl Walter, who then built the Peter Bent Brigham version of the rotating kidney. The Harvard group with John P. Merrill probably did more for the further propagation of dialysis than any other group."[1] These events produced the machine pictured here. It is a modified version of Kolff's first successful dialyzer and was called the Kolff-Brigham artificial kidney. The modifications to the machine produced at the hospital by Dr. Walter, a surgeon-engineer there, were turned over to the Edward A. Olsen Company of Ashland, Massachusetts, which designed and manufactured it.[2] Dr. Merrill was a major figure in the Brigham group studying and performing dialysis.

In 1950 two physicians who also were captains in the Army Medical Corps, Paul E. Teschan and Marion E. McDowell, were dispatched to Brigham Hospital for dialysis training in anticipation of a future need for it in Washington, D.C., at Walter Reed and on the battlefield in Korea in the war that was beginning there. The artificial kidney in this illustration, with a white-coated Captain Teschan standing on the left, arrived at Walter Reed in Spring 1951 and was used there until March 1952, when it was shipped to the Renal Center of the 11th Evacuation Hospital of the 8th Army in Korea to treat military casualties experiencing acute kidney failure.[3] In a letter from the battlefield to the manufacturer Edward Olsen in November 1952, Teschan observed that the artificial kidney his company had produced worked as well when situated in a Korean rice paddy as in a Washington hospital, and that in the previous month his team had performed an average of one dialysis a day.[4]

Nazi hands a portion of the more than ten thousand men rounded up in Rotterdam by the Nazis to work in Germany. Kolff displayed courage in confronting and persuading the commander of this operation to allow him to choose and take charge of eight hundred men in most serious need of medical attention.[13]

During the war, Kolff produced eight artificial kidneys. Several were sent to other Dutch cities, to which Kolff traveled to treat patients for whom grave illnesses and perilous wartime conditions made transport to Kolff's hospital in Kampen impractical and unwise. Other artificial kidneys were stored in safe places to prevent bombing of the dialysis program. When the war ended, and as soon as transportation was feasible, Kolff shipped three abroad – to the Hammersmith Hospital in London, to the Mount Sinai Hospital in New York, and to the Royal Victoria Hospital in Montreal (Figure 6).[14]

In the postwar period, through lecture tours, correspondence, and his publications, Kolff inspired a worldwide interest in the research, development, and clinical use of the artificial kidney. He created a field of interest by forming its basic technology into a workable instrument, elaborating its technical use, and defining the principles of clinical management and organization needed to care for patients. Kolff was not the first person to attempt kidney dialysis. He neither introduced nor refined some of its essential elements, such as the use of the cellophane membrane or its anticlotting agent heparin. But he made the conceptual, technical, and social connections needed to establish the innovation's usefulness and is therefore the central figure in the development of the artificial kidney.

Until 1960 kidney dialysis was directed largely at treating medical crises in which kidney malfunction imperiled the health and life of a patient, the problem it had been designed to meet. Thus, it was used

---

References: for Figure 6:

1. Kolff, WJ. First Clinical Experience with the Artificial Kidney. *Annals of Internal Medicine.* 1965; 62:615. 2. Edward A. Olsen Company. The Kolff-Brigham Artificial Kidney. Ashland, Mass.: Olsen Company; n.d. Anonymous technical pamphlet published by the Oslen Company, and in the Archives of the National Museum of Health and Medicine, Armed Forces Institute of Pathology, located at the Walter Reed Army Medical Center, Washington, D.C. 3. Notes on Artificial Kidney Machine (Rotating Drum) at Walter Reed General Hospital. Unattributed and undated two-page document in the archives of ibid. 4. Letter from Captain Paul E. Teschan to Mr. Edward A. Olsen, November 4, 1952. It exists as a page from an unattributed publication and is located in the archives of ibid.

mainly to remove the buildup in the blood of ingested toxic substances or overdoses of ordinary drugs such as aspirin, of physiological body chemicals that during illness could accumulate to dangerous levels such as potassium, and of urea and other waste products resulting from damaged kidneys. The danger and pain of reconnecting the blood vessels of patients to the dialysis machine repeatedly over long periods of time restricted the use of dialysis to short-term interventions. But even its brief application was limited by the need of hospitals to have a team of physicians, nurses, and technicians available during the day to treat admitted patients and on call at all times to deal with emergencies.

However, an interest in expanding the usefulness of the dialysis machine by expanding the length of time over which it could be used drew the attention of Paul E. Teschan. Teschan was an army physician who in 1950 had received training to use an artificial kidney and was sent to staff hospital units treating soldiers with kidney failure in Washington, D.C., and abroad during the Korean War (see note to Figure 6). In the late 1950s, he advocated the routine use of the artificial kidney to prevent the kidney failure common in burn patients, and he called the method prophylactic dialysis. But his efforts to keep tubes connected to blood vessels as access sites for repeated dialysis did not work because of shortcomings of design and materials.[15] Still, the challenge to do more with the kidney machine stirred others to engage the problem. Success would come from the American Northwest.

At this time, Belding Scribner was a physician in charge of a small dialysis center at the University of Washington at Seattle and had been involved with the therapy for a decade. In the late 1950s, he became particularly upset when one of his patients, whom dialysis had temporarily rescued from kidney failure, died for lack of a long-term treatment. For weeks after his patient's death, Scribner dwelt on the problem. Then one night he awoke from sleep with the solution. A U-shaped tube (or shunt) connected to tubes placed permanently in an artery and vein of the patient's arm would allow blood to circulate between them, could be removed for a dialysis hookup, and reinserted afterward. Thus without the need to constantly repuncture blood vessels, long-term dialysis would be possible. But he faced the technical issue of finding a material for his device that did not cause clots when the patient's blood passed over its surface. A chance collegial encounter, typical of the way that ideas are generated in university environments, provided an answer. Loren Winterscheid, a young surgeon with whom Scribner conversed in a stairwell, suggested that Teflon, a material just introduced onto the market, might do the job. Scribner consulted an engineer, Wayne Quinton, who worked with him to develop a shunt whose nonstick Teflon surface prevented clotting. This shunt and its modifications kept the first patient on whom it was used, Clyde Shields, alive for eleven years, and the fifth patient, Tim Albers, for thirty-six. As the physician-journalist Lawrence Altman recounts: "After Dr. Scribner reported his early results in Atlantic City, the audience of researchers stood and cheered – a rarity at a scientific meeting."[16] With this innovation, long-term center-based treatment with the dialysis machine became a reality, and as the 1960s began, medicine and America entered new social, ethical, and political territory.

But it is important to place the introduction of center-based kidney dialysis into the framework of two other treatments for kidney disease that had become available at this time and the challenges of using them. One was home dialysis, which could significantly decrease the costs of care and thus increase the afflicted population's access to effective therapy. In the 1960s advances occurred that reduced the complexity, cost, and user-unfriendliness of home dialysis. Nonetheless, patients needed training in operating the dialysis machine, in monitoring how their body was responding to the procedure, and in performing therapeutic actions such as taking required drugs. They were responsible as well for identifying relatives or friends who could respond readily to emergencies created by the dialysis process. Many patients found these actions too difficult to contemplate or meet. Medical experts also believed that the system to deliver home dialysis needed refinement, and the level of stress associated with bringing long-term, life-sustaining therapy into the home required greater study. A second alternative was a natural kidney through transplantation. At this time, the effectiveness of kidney transplantation was growing, made possible by the earliest long-term and successful transplant, which occurred at the Peter Bent Brigham Hospital in Boston in 1954 and used the kidney of one twin to save the other. Yet transplantation was still in its infancy, and its recipients faced a physically daunting, expensive, and continuing battle with the efforts of the body to reject and destroy the foreign substance that the kidney represented. A 1971 study comparing the length of survival of those treated with these three therapies for chronic kidney disease ranked dialysis provided in centers first, dialysis given in homes second, and transplants from cadaver organs (their most common source) last.[17]

Thus, in the 1960s center-based dialysis was the most advanced and common form of this care. But its use led the United States into its first peacetime encounter with a new feature of modern technological medicine – deciding how to ration a scarce and costly resource among the many claimants for it.

Scribner's initial success with Clyde Shields and the several other patients he worked with in the early investigative phase of long-term dialysis convinced him not only of the need to continue the work to improve the technology but also to devise an organization suited to deal with the dilemma produced by its success. New patients brought into the program would not necessarily replace older ones, after the model of acute-care medicine in which hospital beds were turned over quickly. Instead, new patients would join older ones, whose survival depended typically on twelve-hour, twice-weekly dialysis sessions that continued as long as they lived. The problem of chronic care was accommodating the medical and social needs of a cohort of patients whose growing size was linked to the achievements of their treatment. This meant having an adequate number of dialyzers; a staff of competent doctors, nurses, social workers, and technicians; administrators sensitive to the challenges of work at an innovative frontier; and the financial resources to pay for it all. Indeed, it soon became clear that this cost would be a minimum of $10,000 a year per patient.[18] It was out of the reach of most people to afford medical care at this level.

Such factors caused Scribner to suggest that the Kings County Medical Society in Seattle take the lead in creating a separate, nonprofit institution to administer a dialysis program for community members with chronic kidney failure, an idea that led to the establishment of the Seattle Artificial Kidney Center. The center recognized from the start the enormity of a basic problem it had to face: how many and which patients should have access to its care, which would be given at the Swedish Hospital of Seattle? The center's staff felt, rightly, that having taken the responsibility to treat a patient, the center remained obligated to that person for as long as care was needed, which could mean to the end of the patient's life. This imperative placed a tremendous burden on the center to develop the right selection process.

Scribner and others decided that such circumstances favored the presence of the community in rationing choices that involved its members. In the end, the center developed a three-stage process. The Medical Advisory Committee would choose from prospective patients whose biological, clinical, and psychological status made them good candidates to tolerate the stress, infections, and uncertainties of long-term dialysis. The profiles of medically acceptable candidates would then be given to a group of seven laypeople, the Admissions Advisory Committee, whose job was to develop and use social criteria to select who would be treated. Its recommendation was transmitted to the center's medical director and the Executive Committee of its board for final approval.

The number of patients chosen was largely determined by the center's ability to gain financial support. Its staff worked hard and creatively to find resources. They lobbied foundations, insurance companies, and the government for resources and were fairly successful. Still, four years after its creation, the center could afford to have but twenty-one people under treatment, losing only three of the patients who had enrolled in the program. The limited number of available places thus sorely tested the selection process.[19]

Six months before the center opened, in the summer of 1961, the Admissions Advisory Committee met to establish, with the help of other center representatives, criteria on which to base decisions. The group included a banker, a homemaker, a government official, a minister, a lawyer, a labor leader, and a surgeon. The Medical Advisory Committee suggested, through two of its members present at the meeting, that the group adopt an age criterion that excluded older people, who presented the problem of medical risk, and younger people, who posed problems of cooperation and ability to tolerate the medical regimen of the treatment, such as its strict diet. In the end, age limits were set: initially at twenty-five to forty-five years but later expanded from seventeen to fifty years. The two medical representatives also offered to sit in on committee sessions as advisers, an offer the committee accepted.

At subsequent meetings other criteria were developed. The changing and limited resources of the center led it from the beginning to expect patients to share responsibility for the cost of dialysis. While its magnitude waxed and waned, by the mid-1960s it was pegged at about 30 percent. Thus, the Admissions Advisory Committee agreed to have financial ability as a criterion.

A geographic standard was also established. The argument was made that resources and funds raised by the local community for the scientific and clinical effort that created the Seattle center justified confining its benefits to its donors – the residents of Washington State. (Later the area was enlarged to include the Northwest region of Washington, Oregon, Montana, Idaho, and Alaska.) Other allocation criteria specified by the committee included marital status; number of dependents; emotional stability, which was a factor in evaluating ability to gain from the therapy; occupation, including past performance and future potential; and references by others who knew the candidate. The combined criteria of patient selection ultimately settled on by the Admissions Advisory and Medical Advisory Committees were summarized as follows:

- Stable, emotional mature, responsible citizen
- Absence of long-standing hypertension and permanent complications
- Demonstrated willingness to cooperate
- Age (seventeen to fifty years "physiologically")
- Slow deterioration of renal function (creatinine 8–12 mg %)
- Six months' residence in area
- Financial support
- Value to community
- Potential for rehabilitation
- Psychological and psychiatric compatibility[20]

Finally, the Admissions Advisory Committee members decided to keep their own identities and the patients they evaluated anonymous.

It did not take long for the general public to learn of these events in Seattle. In 1962, shortly after the kidney center began to function, a feature story in *Life* magazine that focused on the Seattle selection process appeared and captured the attention of the nation. The article's riveting title was "They Decide Who Lives, Who Dies." It provided an in-depth view of the reasoning and feelings of ordinary people involved in life-in-the-balance decisions.[21]

Its author, Shana Alexander, viewed the artificial kidney as the harbinger of a new era in which changing failed body parts with mechanical ones had become a reality, and she was right. While in past centuries artificial limbs had replaced arms and legs, never before were the functions of a life-sustaining organ assumed over the long term by a machine. She described the artificial kidney as a "medical laundromat" and drew readers into the story of its use through the experience of a real patient, depicting his spare diet (cornstarch mixtures, vegetables, and fruit); his feelings during biweekly, twelve-hour hookups to the machine (he often felt a prisoner of the system), and his journey from near death to near normality.

However, the heart of the tale was the deliberations of the Admissions Advisory Committee, which she called the "Life or Death Committee." She describes its seven members and the personal accounts of their journey through uncharted ethical territory. She also persuades them to construct from their memories a facsimile of an actual committee meeting, convened to fill two open dialysis slots from a list of five candidates, all in equally urgent need of care. In this dialogue, we see them comparing the merits of a housewife (she had only two children and was unlikely to settle in Seattle for treatment), an aircraft worker with six children (having a low recovery potential), an accountant and a chemist (having the highest education of the candidates and thus better able to serve society), and a small-business man with three children and active in his church (an attribute thought to show the strong character and moral purpose helpful in meeting the challenges of dialysis).[22] They end up choosing the aircraft worker and the small-business man, the patient who is profiled in the story.

Alexander also interviewed each committee member and found them daunted by the prospect of comparing lives and deciding worth: "In theory," says the lawyer, "I believe that a man's contribution to society should determine our ultimate decision. But I'm not so doggone sure that a great painting or a symphony would loom larger in my own mind than the needs of a woman with six children." The members express uncertainty about making such decisions and a concern about the inadequacy of their experience and knowledge for the rationing task. Some felt their function was to remove pressure from the doctors by taking over the allocation judgments. Several believed that the experimental dimension of treatment through an artificial kidney gave them ethical leeway, that the patients not selected would die whether or not they were chosen for dialysis. Others brought up problems with the evidence they used to make selections. They worried about making critical decisions without adequate data, and about choosing life or death for others "on a virtually intuitive basis," as the state official put it. The surgeon, the only professional committee member, who indicated that he served not as doctor but as citizen, revealed that, at its first meeting, the committee considered drawing straws as the selection process but rejected this chance-based solution in favor of examining candidates from a comprehensive perspective of their past and their prospects. As the labor leader put it, "If the Seattle trial is to be a pilot for other communities, we cannot afford any human failures. Also, we haven't got the funds. So I want to pick the man with the most *will power*, the fellow who is least likely to give up.... That's why knowing about a candidate's past life would rate so heavily with me – it's an indication of *character*."[23]

Alexander was skeptical about a selection process that required committee members to choose by comparing lives. She wondered whether the person making the greatest contribution to society or the one leaving it with the greatest burden would be the most worth saving under the committee's criteria. On the basis of its decisions, she mused that a prospective dialysis candidate would be "well-advised to father a great many children, then throw away all his money."[24] Her skepticism was shared by Willem Kolff, who also was troubled by the social criteria embedded in the Seattle admission standards. He noted that the previously discussed first patient whom his dialysis machine had saved after the war was sixty-seven, not considered by him or others a "useful" member of society, and indeed admitted to his hospital from a prison in which Dutch supporters of national socialism were detained. "Many of our fellow citizens would have accepted her death without regret," wrote Kolff. "May those who decide whether a certain patient should be admitted to a dialysis center in the year 1965 remember that the physician's primary responsibility is toward the patient."[25]

In 1968 a law review article portrayed the selection process as "a disturbing picture of the bourgeoisie sparing the bourgeoisie, of the Seattle Committee measuring persons with its own middle-class suburban value system: scouts, Sunday school, Red Cross. This rules out creative non-conformists. . . . The Pacific Northwest is no place for a Henry David Thoreau with bad kidneys."[26] By this time, there were 121 long-term dialysis centers in the United States. All used a medical evaluation in making their choices, and some used psychiatric, social worth, or financial criteria in a decision process involving medical or lay committees, or both.[27] Thus, the Seattle model of choosing dialysis candidates had spread to other centers.

The main problem raised by the Seattle selection procedure was its effort to judge the lives of people. It did this in two ways. First, it made value to community an explicit standard for admission. Second, it introduced social factors to evaluate a candidate's ability to benefit from dialysis, which is perilous because benefits discussions that incorporate such factors can easily slide to a focus on whether one patient or another deserves the therapy more. The overall effect of applying social standards to rationing decisions in Seattle was the turning of committee judgments into personal commentaries on who had led the better life, who was more needed or valuable to others, and who had displayed appealing virtues.

The allocation process used by the Seattle kidney center provides important lessons, one of which is to recognize the social context in which its decision making occurred. For the Seattle effort was a pioneering peacetime attempt to ration costly medical resources with neither guiding precedents nor the presence of a robust and public ethics discourse to focus its reasoning. These limitations should be recognized in considering the committee's procedures and choices.

The small number of people treated at the dialysis centers by the mid-1960s (about 800) plus the even fewer treated through transplantation (273 worldwide from March 1964 to March 1965) were a fraction of those needing such care. A 1965 analysis projected that 5–10,000 new patients each year in the United States needed dialysis, for whom at least twenty thousand dialysis machines would have to be available on a geographic basis.[28] One fact about dealing with long-term kidney failure was now clear to its advocates: the numerical disparity between those receiving and those left out of care, as well as the controversy generated by the dialysis selection process, were no longer products of technological shortcomings but of financial constraint. Even if a superior therapy could be developed, most people who suffered from failing kidneys could not afford it.

This reality was depicted in a 1967 article in the magazine *Redbook*. Unlike the 1962 *Life* article, which concentrated on the dialysis selection process and on the fortunate outcome of a person accepted for it, the *Redbook* story told of a fruitless search for therapy and ultimately of death. Its focus was a twenty-five-year-old scientist, who came to Washington, D.C., in 1962 with his wife, young son, a newly gained doctoral degree, and a job in research. Soon after settling in, he consulted doctors about symptoms that turned out to be signs of chronic kidney failure. He learned that his only long-term hope was access to an artificial kidney. His wife then embarked on a vigorous campaign to get treatment for her husband, a quest made more difficult because he had diabetes, which increased his risk of complications on dialysis. She encountered problems. Officials at Washington hospitals told her dialyzers in the area and the trained technicians to run them were in short supply, and the cost of such care was $10,000 a year. The medical and financial struggle of the couple was ended by the husband's death four years after he fell sick with kidney failure. The director of a midwestern hospital described a nationwide problem, which this case epitomized: "We have a kidney machine, but only one technician who knows how to work it. If she is sick, we are helpless. Frankly, we are unable to help long-term patients who have completely lost the natural use of their kidneys. We keep our machine for emergencies – poisoning cases and so on."[29]

Only one national institution with the resources and political power to meet this problem existed, the federal government. During the mid-1960s, it began to focus on kidney failure. Powerful legislators spoke out, among them Senator Henry Jackson: "It's a terrible thing that probably several thousand men and women will die this year and next who might be saved by an artificial kidney if equipment were available and skilled technicians at hand."[30] The Veterans Administration started to place dialysis units in its hospitals across the country, the National Institutes of Health created research programs on kidney dialysis and transplantation, the Public Health Service made grants to establish dialysis centers, and the Bureau of the Budget convened an expert committee to write a report on all aspects of the issue. Named after its chair Carl Gottschalk and issued in 1967, the report resolved the debate on whether dialysis and transplantation were experimental or standard therapies in favor of the standard side, which justified and increased their use for kidney failure.[31]

Alongside this official activity, influential private-sector voices entered the scene politically, anchored by Belding Scribner of the Seattle Artificial Kidney Center and George Schreiner, a leading kidney expert at Georgetown University and president and later chair of the legislative committee of the National Kidney Foundation. Together with congressional allies, they secured greater federal funding to treat kidney failure so that, by 1972, about 10,000 people were on dialysis. These actions collectively generated considerable local and national press coverage about the potential of long-term kidney therapy and set the stage for groundbreaking federal legislation.[32]

During 1972 Congress was considering a bill extending the 1965 Medicare law insuring people over the age of sixty-five to cover disabled people below this age. Supporters of kidney disease funding sponsored an amendment to classify its sufferers as disabled and thus included under the umbrella of the legislation. At hearings on the issue testimony was given by a dialysis patient and member of the National Association of Patients on Hemodialysis, Nathan Glazer:

I am 43 years old, married for 20 years, with two children ages 14 and 10. I was a salesman until a couple of months ago until it became necessary for me to supplement my income to pay for the dialysis supplies. I tried to sell a non-competitive line, was found out, and was fired. Gentlemen, what should I do? End it all and die? Sell my house for which I worked so hard, and go on welfare? Should I go into the hospital under my hospitalization policy, then I cannot work? Please tell me. If your kidneys failed tomorrow, wouldn't you want the opportunity to live? Wouldn't you want to see your children grow up?"[33]

In addition to making his statement, Glazer received permission from the House Ways and Means Committee to be dialyzed in the hearing room in front of committee members. The treatment lasted five minutes and was declared by them as "excellent testimony." Perhaps excellent but indeed perilous. Some of his physician colleagues worried that a serious adverse event incurred during dialysis could threaten their cause. He did in fact experience a very rapid heartbeat, but the dialysis was quickly stopped and the problem went unrecognized by the committee.[34]

Victory came in the fall of 1972. Congress passed and the president signed legislation that included a provision declaring that patients with chronic kidney disease who needed dialysis or transplantation were disabled for purposes of payment under Medicare, which covered most of the costs of therapy. No longer did patients with kidney failure need to face selection committees or certain death from lack of funds. Political will and technological advance had joined to hold a mortal disease at bay. The chair of the Senate committee that considered the legislation, Russell Long, encapsulated societal attitudes toward patients with kidney disease and congressional views about the bill that produced its passage:

I can recall testimony by a doctor that impressed me. He testified that he had patients with kidney failure – hardworking people, good, responsible citizens, honest, salt-of-the-earth people. "What are my possibilities?" they would ask. "Kidney transplant, dialysis, or death," he would reply. "What does it cost?" was their next question. When told, they responded, "There is no way to raise that kind of money. What am I to do?" ... I sat there and thought to myself: We are the greatest nation on earth, the wealthiest per capita. Are we so hard pressed that we cannot pay for this? A life could be extended 10 to 15 years. You're not going to make any money that way. But it struck me as a case of compelling need.[35]

This legislation made chronic kidney disease at that time the only illness whose diagnosis triggered a federal entitlement to care. The widespread, drama-filled publicity generated by withholding such technology from those whose lives it could save produced an unstoppable political tide favoring governmental intervention. What is more, the artificial kidney delivered to the public the news that a new technological medicine had arrived, one that would be hard to afford, difficult to allocate among those who needed its help, and would require innovative concepts and policies to control.

Almost a half-century has elapsed since the start of the 1960s when the artificial kidney became a prominent feature of the medical and public landscape. During this time society and medicine searched without success for adequate responses to the challenge of wisely applying and broadly providing high technology care. However as the effort proceeded, the staggering cost of technological medicine surpassed not only the resources of individuals to afford but seriously strained the financial capacity of society and its insurance mechanisms to bear. From 1960 to 2006, health care expenditures increased by an average of 2.5 percent per year more than the increase of America's gross domestic product (GDP), which accounts for health care's rising share of the GDP. Indeed from consuming about one of every twenty dollars spent on goods and services in the United States in 1960, health care spending rose to some one in six dollars by 2006 – a path of growth that is unsustainable because of its increasing conflict with other significant national obligations. Studies exploring the causes of this spending rise reach the broadly similar conclusion that technological change in medical practice is the predominent source, accounting for between half to two-thirds of the increase. This is far more than other significant drivers of spending such as increased insurance coverage (from ten to thirteen percent), or personal income growth (between five to twenty percent).[36]

Technological medicine thus is a paradox – at once a savior and a threat. To meet the complexity of using and governing it therefore requires not just innovative social policies, but also fathoming the ethical dimensions of using technology, and understanding basic medical thinking about the nature of health and illness that operates beneath the surface of the health care system, influencing the invention and application of technologies and driving medical judgments, actions, and priorities. The discussion of these matters begun in this and earlier chapters will be carried into subsequent ones.

4

PROMISING RESCUE, PREVENTING RELEASE
The Double Edge of the Artificial Respirator

In 1958 Pope Pius XII publicly responded to a plea for moral guidance from Dr. Bruno Haid, an Austrian physician in charge of the resuscitation service of his hospital. Using techniques anchored by a new generation of more effective artificial respirators, the service had successfully treated people whose breathing had been compromised by accidents or illness. The quandary was this: what to do when, after being saved from dying and sustained by the respirator for weeks or months, some patients didn't recover but lay suspended in a void between life and death? Acknowledging the complexity of the problem, the pope was unsure he could help but offered to try. The exchange between a medical and a religious figure and the landmark response it prompted began an extraordinary medical and societal journey into the promise and danger of new technology. The central controversy engendered by the breathing machine was different from the one that enveloped the artificial kidney. With the kidney, the perplexing issue was the quandary of access; with the respirator, it became the demand for release.

The emergency produced when a person stops breathing has evoked inventions to bring air into the lungs in one of two basic ways: forcing air into them at above atmospheric pressure, with so-called positive pressure devices, or creating a partial vacuum around the chest, whose expansion caused air to enter and inflate them, with so-called negative pressure devices. Some later machines combined both types of pressure.

A bellows was the first positive pressure device used to bring air to the lungs. In the sixteenth century, the anatomist Andreas Vesalius described an experiment on an animal whose life he maintained with a bellows through which he applied intermittent positive pressure to inflate the lungs.[1] By the nineteenth century, squads charged with the rescue of drowning victims used a bellows connected to the windpipe by a tube through which air was forced into the lungs. But the combined assault of the air pulses and the problematic tubal connection produced more damage than relief. In 1825 the Royal Humane Society of England declared the bellows and tube unsafe and recalled them from use. To moderate the destructive power of the bellows, a model appeared that placed gradations on its handle. This allowed users to blow a volume of air into the lungs proportionate to the size of the patient. But it did not improve the resuscitative effectiveness of the technology.[2]

Parallel to efforts to create successful positive pressure devices were ones to invent machines that used negative pressure. Their basic design was an airtight container that enveloped the body from the neck down. Pumping air from the container lowered the atmospheric pressure within it. This caused the rib cage to enlarge and consequently air to flow into the lungs – the equivalent of events that naturally produce inhalation. When the pressure was returned to the normal atmospheric level, the lungs naturally contracted and accomplished exhalation. Such events needed to occur intermittently to mimic normal breathing. Several mid-nineteenth-century inventors created ventilators based on this concept, but their designs and operation made them ineffective in saving lives.[3] In the twentieth century, the needs of surgery stimulated the search for effective techniques to maintain the breathing of patients.[4] More aggressive and complicated operations were being undertaken that placed great stress on breathing. To deal with this expanding surgical activity, an unusual and complicated invention appeared in 1904. It was a room-sized ventilator and operating space whose pressure was continuously kept below the normal atmospheric level and in which assembled the surgeons, their assistants, and the body of the patient. The main feature of its design required the head of the patient, whose neck was embraced by an airtight collar, to extend through a wall into an adjoining room. The patient's head thus was exposed to higher pressure than the patient's chest, and this pressure difference facilitated breathing.[5] But the technique was cumbersome to the conducting of surgery and, after several decades of popularity, was abandoned. Further, no solution had been developed for patients requiring longer-term ventilation.

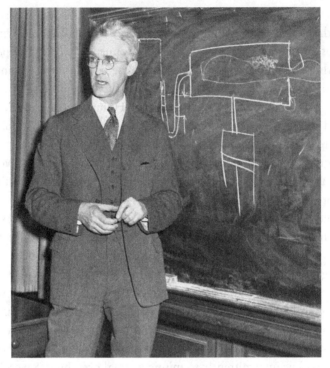

Figure 7. Philip Drinker and a chalkboard drawing of a respirator (ca. 1930). Courtesy of the Children's Hospital Boston Archives, Boston, Massachusetts.

This posed a significant dilemma in the late 1920s, when effective ventilators with a capacity for extended use were vital to help victims of the poliomyelitis epidemics that were circling the world. The disease could immobilize the muscles that produced respiration and endanger the lives of its victims. It was especially threatening to society because of the large number of children it attacked. Responding to this challenge, physicians at the Children's Hospital in Boston sought the aid of Philip Drinker, an engineer at the Harvard School of Public Health, to create a technology that sustained the breathing of polio victims long enough to give their bodies time to recover and take over the task (Figure 7). Drinker visited the Children's Hospital and witnessed the struggle of its young patients, described in telling comments by the pediatrician J. L. Wilson: "Of all the experiences the physician must undergo, none can be more distressing than to watch respiratory paralysis in a child with poliomyelitis – to watch him become more and more dyspneic [air hungry], using with increasing vigor every available muscle of neck, shoulder and chin – silent, wasting no breath for speech, wide-eyed, and frightened, conscious almost to the last breath."[6]

Drinker accepted the challenge to produce a ventilator and asked a physiologist and colleague, Louis Shaw, to join the effort. Shaw's scientific work on respiration in cats gave him experience in using a small airtight box that enclosed the cat's body but left the head of the animal extended outside. They designed a respirator using such a box and a combination of negative and positive pressure to run it. Experiments with anesthetized animals showed the apparatus capable of giving prolonged and successful ventilation. Now they were ready to leave the laboratory and build a human-sized version, useful not only in polio but also in other respiratory calamities, like drowning and electric shock. For this they developed a tank-shaped machine that alternatively produced negative and positive pressure. Two vacuum-cleaner motors powered the first model, which was made in 1927 (Figure 8). A second model (in 1928) was used in the first clinical trial of their invention. In the autumn of that year, it maintained the breathing of an eight-year-old polio victim for 122 hours, a duration that had never been achieved before. Unfortunately, she died of complications from the disease. But in 1929 a respirator with improvements saved the life of a woman suffering from an accidental drug overdose; and a college student stricken with polio who had remained on the machine for several weeks, was gradually weaned from it, and returned to normal life.[7]

The respiratory treatment required by polio victims was different from that of other conditions. Previous breathing devices were applied mainly to emergency situations like drowning or to patients having surgery. Their needs could be attained by sustaining respiration from several minutes to several hours. Polio victims could need days, weeks, or longer-term support. The innovation by Drinker and Shaw ultimately met this demand. Drinker and a medical colleague Charles McKhann summarized the requirements of a respirator for illnesses like polio: "To prove satisfactory, such an apparatus must be capable of working steadily over a long period of time; it must be adaptable to individuals of various ages and sizes; it must be so constructed that the rate and depth of respiration can be controlled; lastly, and most important, it

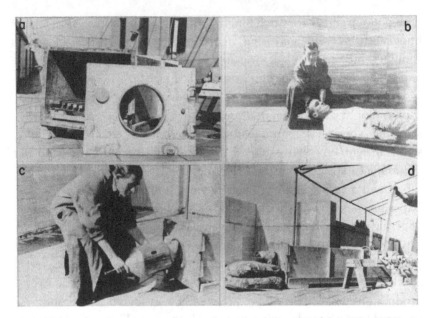

Figure 8. Construction and demonstration of an early iron lung. Courtesy of The Children's Hospital Boston Archives, Boston, Massachusetts.

This is the first Drinker-Shaw respirator, made in mid-1927. They described it as "consisting of a cheap galvanized metal box, with bed made from 'garage creepers' and two household vacuum cleaners with hand-operated valve as the source of alternative positive and negative pressure."[1] The scientists were funded by the Consolidated Gas Company of New York, which was interested in the practical possibilities of long-term artificial respiration because its rescue squads frequently treated patients with breathing problems caused by carbon monoxide poisoning, electric shock, drowning, and so forth. Experiments with people not suffering from such conditions convinced Drinker and Shaw that their technology could have medical uses.

Reference: 1. Drinker P, Shaw LA. The Prolonged Administration of Artificial Respiration. *Journal of the Franklin Institute*. 1932; 213:358.

must be capable of producing adequate artificial respiration without discomfort or harm to the patient."[8] The name *iron lung* was quickly attached to the machine.[9]

Subsequent use of the iron lung produced mixed results. A study of polio cases at the Children's Hospital in Boston during the early 1930s found it far more effective in treating patients with paralysis of muscles associated with breathing (eighteen of twenty-three survived on the iron lung) than in those who had the more severe bulbar type of polio affecting connections between the brain and spinal cord (seven of twenty recovered), a finding confirmed by subsequent investigations. However, as the device became more widely applied, some

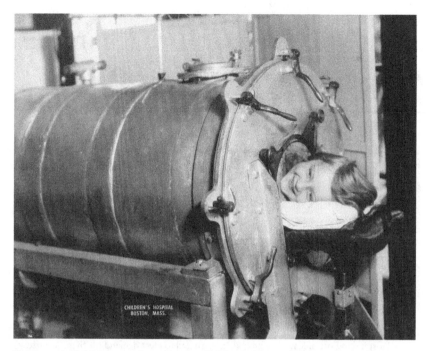

Figure 9. A child in a respirator at the Children's Hospital, Boston (ca. early 1930s). Courtesy of the Children's Hospital Boston Archives, Boston, Massachusetts.

clinicians reported dismal outcomes in treating all types of polio (Figures 9 and 10).[10]

Disparities in outcome such as this are common when new and complicated technologies are introduced into practice. The iron lung required perceptive decision making by physicians in prescribing the care for the patient on it, critical judgments by nurses in giving the actual hour-to-hour care necessary to preserve the patient's life, and the ability of clinical services such as the laboratories and the hospital administration itself to cope with the problems of managing long-term critical care. In some hospitals such teamwork was simply better than in others. The success of technologies like iron lungs thus depends not only on their intrinsic mechanical effectiveness but also on the capabilities of the organizations that house them.

Two problems proved particularly difficult for doctors who treated polio patients in the 1930s, the first decade of the iron lung's widespread use. One was a fear that, after placing patients on the machine, they would retain lifelong dependence on it. In fact, weaning patients from

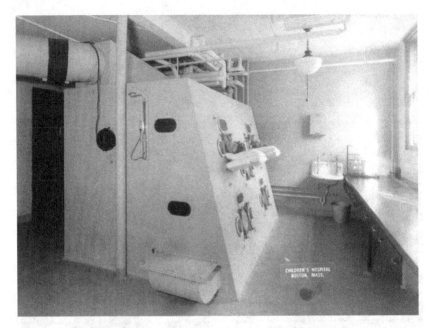

Figure 10. A room-sized respirator (supporting the breathing of two patients) at the Children's Hospital in Boston (ca. early 1930s), constructed to meet demand for them. Courtesy of the Children's Hospital Boston Archives, Boston, Massachusetts.

Intensive attention by nurses was necessary to maintain patients in iron lungs. To keep them clean, monitor vital functions, apply hot packs to painful muscles, turn them over to prevent skin sores, or give intravenous fluids could take the combined efforts of two to four nurses. This care was given through the ports in the respirator, which were surrounded by rubber disks to maintain pressure inside it. The insertion of nurses' arms and materials into the respirator was made during expiratory phase of breathing, so that the seal could be maintained during inspiration.[1]

Reference: 1. Snider GL. Thirty Years of Mechanical Ventilation: Changing Implications. *Archives of Internal Medicine.* 1983; 143:745.

the machines could sometimes prove very difficult. This led some physicians to delay the decision on whether to start iron-lung therapy and thereby jeopardize their patients' chances for recovery.[11] The other problem was scarcity, for at times there were fewer iron lungs than patients who needed them. This forced hospital physicians to ration the machine and deal with the question, Should it be given to the sickest patient with the poorest chance to survive or to the one with less severe symptoms but more likely to respond to the therapy? Unlike the lengthy artificial kidney selection process weighted with social criteria, whose claimants had a chronic illness and usually could wait out the process, polio victims needed urgent care. This produced rapid physician choices based not on societal issues but on physical determinants and the doctor's general view of which circumstance was more ethically compelling: a greater threat to life or greater chance to recover. The scarcity of respiratory technology also led some physicians to justify removing a patient from the iron lung and giving it to another who was more critically ill.[12]

In part, the shortage of iron lungs was based on expense. The machines of the 1930s initially cost about $2,500 but soon came down to $1,000. Because of the price, some hospitals did not buy machines until the appearance of a polio epidemic. However, without a trained staff to use the device, just having it on the premises could not guarantee good outcomes. Further, the cost of hospital care was burdensome to families, and insurance to cover expenses was unavailable. But in 1938 the National Foundation for Infantile Paralysis was founded by the most famous victim of the illness, President Franklin Roosevelt. It launched a nationwide effort to support research and help families of polio patients care and pay for treatment, anchored by the annual March of Dimes campaigns. Between 1938 and 1962, the foundation raised about $630 million to support its work. The foundation funded research efforts, disseminated public information about hospitals able to provide polio care, lent respiratory equipment to cities without the adequate technology to confront a polio epidemic, instituted training programs for hospital personnel in respiratory care, and created special centers to treat chronically disabled patients.[13,14] These efforts meliorated the need to ration iron lungs.

From the 1930s through the 1940s, a highly significant two-track process of innovation occurred in respiratory care. The treatment of poliomyelitis was centered on the combination of negative and positive pressure therapy provided by the iron lung. At the same time, anesthetists in the operating room, who could not use respiratory techniques that wrapped their patients in tanks, were developing ventilation techniques to support patients based on the intermittent positive pressure ventilation (IPPV) idea, historically expressed in the use of the bellows. However, now better techniques of connecting the machine to the patient's windpipe and other improvements to introduce air into the lungs made IPPV a critical part of standard practice in European and American operating rooms. Essentially, the worlds of the clinic and the operating room developed and used separate means of meeting the respiratory problems of patients. The 1952 epidemic of polio in Copenhagen dramatically merged this bipolar world.

In August 1952 a new wave of polio swept through Copenhagen, whose most seriously ill patients were sent to the Blegdam Hospital, the center for treating communicable diseases. The first thirty-one admitted patients received standard treatment including tank-type ventilation. Twenty-seven of them died, in part from ventilation ineffectiveness and from shortage – the hospital had only seven ventilators. Facing the imminent death of the twenty-eighth patient, H. C. A. Lassen, chief physician in the communicable diseases department, called Bjørn Ibsen, the senior anesthetist of the hospital, to consult on alternative therapy for the patient. They made the decision to apply measures anesthetists routinely used in operating rooms to maintain breathing for patients having surgery. Thus, they treated the polio victim with IPPV created by manually compressing an anesthesia bag in synchrony with the breathing efforts of the patient, introduced air into the lungs via a cuffed tube inserted through a surgical opening in the windpipe, and removed excess lung secretions through it. The patient improved dramatically and was returned to the iron-lung-type ventilator (a shell called a cuirass respirator enclosing the chest and abdomen) on which she had first been placed. She declined rapidly, was removed, and was restarted on manual IPPV ventilation. She improved again, making clear the need for IPPV treatment over the long term.

The finding initiated a remarkable medical undertaking. As growing numbers of polio patients entered the hospital, the staff faced the dilemma of having found a therapy for polio that was highly effective and lifesaving but whose use demanded an extraordinary effort from and unprecedented numbers of medical personnel. At one point in the epidemic the hospital had nine hundred polio patients, seventy-five of whom needed ventilation on the same day. To do this required 250 medical students for the continuous manual ventilation, 260 nurses at the bedside of patients to meet associated medical needs, and 27 hospital workers to deal with technical problems. To gain the services of the Copenhagen medical students, most of whom were needed for this work, all classes at the medical school were suspended until the epidemic ended.[15]

Critical to the success of the entire operation were the anesthetists. They were assigned to deliver around-the-clock care on each of the three wards where the polio patients were treated. They oversaw the making of windpipe incisions, ensured that the medical students were properly ventilating patients, and gave general respiratory care to the patients. In doing these tasks, they worked cooperatively with the other physicians on the staff. The outcome of the effort was impressive. The mortality rate from polio at the Blegdam Hospital in Copenhagen dropped from more than 80 percent to about 40 percent under this treatment,[16] a statistic confirmed and even lowered in later studies of IPPV use at the bedside.[17]

The Copenhagen crisis transformed respiratory therapy. Machines that effectively delivered automatic IPPV were developed and rapidly spread across Europe, replacing iron-lung technology in treating polio. This diffusion was slower in the United States, where internists who were not familiar with IPPV were in charge of respiratory care, as opposed to anesthetists in Europe who had left the operating room and entered the world of clinical practice to treat victims of polio.[18] The European anesthetists soon extended their scope of care to respiratory crises in general, which had as one result the 1958 petition to the pope to help an anesthetist with a moral crisis.

Dr. Bruno Haid, chief of the anesthesia section of the surgical clinic at the University of Innsbruck in Austria, wrote the pope for ethical guidance about a dilemma created by the newly achieved success of his specialty. It was the problem of what to do when, after a slight improvement, the status of some patients rescued from death with the new technology remained stationary and only automatic artificial respiration kept them alive.

The pope formulated the issues as three sets of questions.[19] First, does one have the right or an obligation to use the new technology of artificial respiration in all cases, even those judged by the treating physicians as hopeless? Second, does one have the right or obligation to remove respiratory technology when, after several days, the patient remains deeply unconscious and if, after being taken away, the circulation of blood will cease in minutes? Allied to this medical problem were religious issues. What to do if the patient has received the last sacraments and the family wishes the life support removed? When, according to the Roman Catholic faith, has death occurred in patients whose life is supported by a respirator? Is the sacrament of extreme unction valid if the heartbeat continues but life depends on the respirator? Third, should a patient made unconscious from brain damage but whose life, manifested by continuing blood circulation, is sustained by artificial respiration and who does not improve after several days be considered biologically or legally dead? Must one wait for the cessation of blood circulation, despite the continuance of artificial respiration, before the patient is considered dead?

Drawing on the church's centuries of reflection on death, the pope dealt with the questions by providing a rationale for using the technology of life support.[20] He declared that those charged with the duty to preserve life and health in cases of serious illness should be held "to use only ordinary means – according to circumstances of persons, places, times and culture – that is to say, means that do not involve any grave burden for oneself or another." A greater obligation would be too burdensome and make it difficult to attain spiritual ends, which he argued were of greater significance than goods such as life, health, and temporal activities. However, people could take more than the strictly necessary measures to maintain life and health if they remained committed to the more important spiritual duties.

Accordingly, the pope advised that neither physicians nor families were obligated to continue the use of artificial respiration technology in cases of illness where deep unconsciousness and/or all hope for recovery was gone. Further, discontinuing the therapy was to be considered an indirect and not the main precipitant of death, even if it caused the circulation of blood to cease. The pope implied it was the illness or accident that caused the death, not the withdrawal of technology. Thus, no moral blame for killing another person could be placed on doctors or family members involved with the decision.

The pope also confronted the issue of when death occurred, since that influenced the validity of extreme unction. In the 1950s cessation of blood circulation medically, legally, and theologically defined the instant when life ended and the soul separated from the body. At that point the patient was no longer a person, a necessary condition to receive the sacraments of the church. But the pope speculated about whether death had taken place when grave brain trauma caused deep unconsciousness and paralysis of respiration function, whose expressions were prevented by the presence of the respirator. He questioned whether a definition of death based on blood circulation could prevail in the face of such new technology. Declaring this an open issue, he nonetheless described a basis for thinking about the essence of life and, in effect, about when death has occurred: "Human life continues for as long as its vital functions – distinguished from the simple life of organs – manifest themselves spontaneously or even with the help of artificial processes."

In this statement, the pope separated the biological from the religious and social self. Human life involved the self-awareness needed to achieve spiritual and other human ends. In the face of machines supporting a body that will never regain the ability to participate in life's endeavors, humans must devise new approaches to comprehending life and death. The sacraments of the church and the decision of families and doctors in these circumstances thus must be performed in the face of doubt.

The pope's concern about the then-current definition of death was well placed, as borne out by a 1959 case report by French physicians. It described a patient in critical condition who had been sustained with artificial respiration for several days before dying. Autopsy revealed an advanced stage of decomposition in the brain: the heart and lungs had continued to function in the face of widespread destruction.[21] During the 1960s, as the ability of technology to sustain life in the face of catastrophic injury or illness grew, anchored and symbolized by the artificial respirator, so did the dilemmas accompanying their use. These included patients trapped in a state of life without awareness; families conflicted about whether to wish for their life or their death and facing, with society, the mounting expense of long-term, technologically intensive care; hospital staff who were emotionally and physically drained from providing care to patients for whom all possibility of recovery had vanished; and hospitals concerned that such patients exhausted their limited financial resources and diverted space that patients able to benefit from treatment could use.

A technological advance from a new field of therapy increased the pressure to revise the criteria of death. In 1954 success was achieved in transplanting a human organ. In a pioneering case noted earlier (see Chapter 3), physicians at Boston's Peter Bent Brigham Hospital transplanted a kidney from a twin to his brother. While a transplant between twins is usually the best biological fit, the ethical problems associated with harvesting an organ from a healthy person, as well as getting enough living donors to meet the demand for transplants, increasingly made cadaver organs the focus of attention. As drugs to prevent organ rejection by the person receiving the transplant and tissue-typing techniques to determine the best donor-recipient biological match grew in effectiveness, all transplantation, but particularly the cadaver-based form, was more successful. In 1966 the one-year survival rate for kidney transplants from living related donors was 70 percent and from cadavers 50 percent.[22] Physicians believed that eventually transplantation would replace dialysis as the long-term solution to kidney failure. It would cost less over time and allow the patient to lead a more normal life without the disruption of regular dialysis. However, transplantation was still in its infancy. In the year ending in March 1965, fewer than three hundred kidneys had been transplanted in the world, and the first heart transplant would occur only in 1967 in South Africa, when Dr. Christiaan Barnard placed a cadaver heart into a dying patient and opened up another frontier for transplantation.[23]

But the use of cadaver transplants required a new concept of death. Taking an organ from a person before death has occurred legally subjected doctors to a wrongful-death action or even to homicide. The difficulty of fixing this time if artificial respiration is maintaining vital organ function is illustrated by a 1963 British case. A young man with multiple skull fractures and brain damage inflicted in a brawl was declared hopelessly injured. When his breathing stopped fourteen hours after admission, artificial respiration was begun and maintained for twenty-four hours, when, with consent from his wife, a kidney was taken for transplant. Then the respirator was removed and no spontaneous breathing or circulation appeared. An inquest to determine the time of death found it had occurred after the kidney was removed. The doctors were criticized but not prosecuted.[24]

Such circumstances caused physicians in the mid-1960s to seek an organ other than the heart whose function would define the existence of life. They turned to the brain. The seminal document of this change emerged from Harvard University in 1968. There, a committee of thirteen faculty members, which included a lawyer, a historian of science, a professor of theology, a biologist, and physicians, convened to examine the matter and defined irreversible coma as a new criterion of death.

They advanced two basic rationales for their recommendation: the multiple problems generated by keeping alive a patient whose heart continued to beat in the face of irreversible brain damage, and freeing the field of organ transplantation from a significant obstacle to its development.

At this time, as the Harvard group noted, *Black's Law Dictionary* characterized death as "the cessation of life; the ceasing to exist; defined by physicians as a total stoppage of the circulation of the blood, and a cessation of the animal and vital functions consequent thereupon, such as respiration, pulsation, etc."[25] The goal of the Harvard report thus was to create a new definition based on signs that a permanently nonfunctioning brain exhibited. It enumerated four: deep coma, which displayed a characteristic electroencephalogram pattern; unawareness of and unresponsiveness to all external stimuli, even those that should produce pain; no muscular movement or breathing (tested on respirator-dependent patients by turning it off three minutes and noting whether they breathed spontaneously) or reflexes such as dilation of the pupils, with light shone into the eye, or blinking; and a flat electroencephalograph, which was recommended but not required to confirm the absence of brain activity. If the doctor in charge and one other medical colleague involved in the case agreed that these criteria were met, death was declared and only then was the respirator turned off. The committee, wisely, emphasized that this action was based on medical criteria, and accordingly, it was "unsound and undesirable to force the family to make the decision." However, if the person were to have organs removed for transplant after the declaration of death, respirator and other artificial support could be applied so that the organs would not deteriorate but remain vital until the patient into whom the organs would be implanted could be gotten to the operating room. Physicians involved in the transplant, the report recommended, should have no involvement in the declaration of death to avoid the appearance of self-interest.

In 1976 the issues raised in the pope's letter and the Harvard committee's report came together in a New Jersey Supreme Court decision in the case of Karen Ann Quinlan. While the social, medical, and legal dimensions of using advanced technologies of rescue like the artificial respirator have been richly elaborated from that time to the present, the Quinlan case was the paradigm for this discourse.

The case began simply but with forebodings of tragedy. On a night in April 1975, Karen Quinlan stopped breathing for at least two fifteen-minute periods while she was with friends. They made efforts at mouth-to-mouth resuscitation and called an ambulance. She arrived at Newton Memorial Hospital in New Jersey, where examining doctors found her unresponsive to stimuli, even deep pain, and with pupils that did not react to light. Subsequent evaluations over the next few days determined that she was in a coma and had suffered brain damage. A respirator was needed to keep her breathing. What may have happened to stop her breathing earlier was not known, but the examining doctor concluded that the oxygen deficit this produced had injured the brain and caused the coma. After some days, Karen was transferred to another New Jersey hospital, where she received more tests and a diagnosis of chronic persistent vegetative state. In this condition, the patient's brain continues to support a number of biological functions such as temperature and blood pressure but loses its ability to respond to the outer or inner environments of life through feeling and thinking. Such a patient has no self-awareness. However, Karen was not brain dead by the Harvard criteria, which requires the loss of both the vegetative and cognitive aspects of brain activity.

But one of the vegetative functions Karen did not have was the ability to breathe on her own, and thus her need for a respirator. It was unclear how long she would live were it removed, but doctors thought such a trial unwarranted because it subjected her to the risk of additional brain damage. However, they agreed on one issue – removing the respirator violated the standards and traditions of medicine. As several months passed, Karen's physical state worsened. She lost considerable weight, assumed a fetal posture, and her limbs were rigid and deformed. She got twenty-four-hour care in the hospital's intensive care unit and was fed through a tube. Her state exposed her to a constant threat of infection. There was neither treatment available to reverse her underlying condition nor hope of restoring her ability to relate to herself or the world.

It was at this stage of Karen's illness, when her doctors felt secure with their grim prognosis, that Karen's family, led by her father, Joseph, requested that the doctors remove her life-supporting technology. The request was made in consultation with his parish priest and the Catholic chaplain of the hospital. For Joseph Quinlan, the concepts proclaimed by Pope Pius XII in his 1958 letter provided the religious and moral justification for his request, without which it was unlikely he would have acted. Mr. Quinlan petitioned a lower court in New Jersey to be made Karen's guardian and given the express power to authorize the discontinuance of her life-supporting technology. When the court refused, Mr. Quinlan appealed the case to the Supreme Court of New Jersey. A brief to the court from the Catholic bishops of New Jersey by Bishop Lawrence Casey on the right to a natural death in cases like that of Karen Quinlan epitomized the interrelation of theology, law, and medicine on the issue:

Each [discipline] must in some way acknowledge the other without denying its own competence. The civil law is not expected to assert a belief in eternal life; nor, on the other hand, is it expected to ignore the right of the individual to profess it, and to form and pursue his conscience in accord with that belief. Medical science is not authorized to directly cause natural death; nor, however, is it expected to prevent it when it is inevitable and all hope of a return to an even partial exercise of human life is irreparably lost. Religion is not expected to define biological death; nor, on its part, is it expected to relinquish its responsibility to assist man in the formation and pursuit of a correct conscience as [by] the acceptance of natural death when science has confirmed its inevitability beyond any hope other than that of preserving biological life in a merely vegetative state."[26]

The court thought that if, by some miracle, Karen could declare how she wished to be treated, given her current condition and prognosis, she would opt to remove the life support even if it meant she would die. It found no compelling state interest that justified requiring Karen to exist as she was, with no chance that she would know herself or the world again. The legal concept of the right to privacy was believed to be broad enough to include under certain conditions a patient's decision to refuse medical treatment, a right whose significance grew as the invasiveness of therapy increased and the prospect of recovery diminished. Supported by a respirator to breathe, around-the-clock intensive care, and faced with the inevitability of bodily decline and death, the strength of the right to privacy for Karen, the court ruled, was greater than the competing state interests either in the preservation and sanctity of life or in defending the right of physicians to provide medical care according to their best judgment. Since Karen could not assert her privacy right, and her wishes could not be determined from conversations or statements she made before being injured, the court designated her father, Joseph, as guardian, with the authority to exercise the right on Karen's behalf.

The court also justified its right to join physicians in decision making in the case, seeing these decisions as reflecting not only medical standards but also community values, an arena where the court had a nondelegatable responsibility. It declared: "The law, equity and justice must not themselves quail and be helpless in the face of modern technological marvels presenting questions hitherto unthought of." While the decision of Karen's doctors to refuse to disconnect life support was consistent with a traditional medical standard to preserve life, the court felt justified in reevaluating the use of this standard as applied to Karen's case. Other pressures affecting medical decisions and the application of medical standards as the threat of malpractice litigation and the possibility of criminal prosecution were recognized, both of which fears the court sought to allay. It wished to help doctors implement the balanced approach to therapy that was central to their work – to not "treat the curable as if they were dying . . . and not treat the hopeless and dying as if they were curable," a balance that the technology of life support had made difficult to sustain.

In addition to hoping that the decisions and discourse in this case would help free doctors from the threat of social and legal coercion so they could ethically exercise medical judgment on behalf of their patients, the court made an important procedural suggestion. It adopted a recommendation found in a 1975 article in the medical literature discussing the value of a multidisciplinary ethics committee, which some hospitals were beginning to form. The committee had representatives from medicine, law, social work, theology, and so forth, and gave physicians a forum in which they could share clinical dilemmas and seek guidance on medical decisions.[27] The court saw the ethics committee as analogous to the multiple-judge panel used by the legal system in the appeals process, in which the value of diffused professional responsibility for decision making was evident. Accordingly, it endorsed the ethics committee as a means of ensuring that difficult judgments were made in conformity with medical standards and not stained by inappropriate motivations of families or physicians. And while emphasizing the helpfulness of these added professional insights in such cases, the court endorsed the usefulness of views from families of incompetent persons.

Thus, it sought to maximize the benefit of its judgments to help doctors deal with the complexities that new technology had introduced in medicine.

Along these lines, it stated unequivocally that, in the Quinlan case, a decision to terminate life support that resulted in Karen's demise would not be homicide "but rather expiration from existing natural causes." It further asserted that even if the termination was thought of as homicide it would not be unlawful, for ending therapy on the basis of the right of privacy in the terms of this case was lawful. Homicide statutes prohibit the unlawful taking of another's life, while the withdrawal of life support was an act of self-determination.

On the basis of these premises, the court formulated its decision. First, by making Karen's father her guardian, it gave him the freedom to choose other physicians for her who could take a decision to remove life support. However, a hospital ethics committee had to be in place with whom the new physicians would consult on the reasonableness of a decision for withdrawing life support from Karen. That having been given, life support could be removed without civil or criminal penalties. The court decision was unanimous, 7–0.

Joseph Quinlan now replaced the physicians treating Karen with new ones. They studied the case and consulted with a newly impanelled hospital ethics committee, which concurred with the decision to remove the central technology, the respirator, which sustained Karen's breathing and life. To the surprise of all, Karen was successfully weaned from the machine. She lived for nearly a decade more in a nursing facility, never regaining consciousness and visited regularly by her family and friends to the end.

The 1958 letter of Pope Pius XII to the Austrian doctor, which initiated contemporary reflection on using life-sustaining technology, has a remarkable resonance with discussions about therapy composed more than 2,500 years ago by Hippocratic physicians. Then medicine was referred to as an art, not a science, and its therapeutic armory was limited. However, the Hippocratics showed why, without a concept of restraint, even modest therapies could wreak great harm. A central document concerned with this issue is one titled *The Art*, which examines the sources of therapeutic power. The power resides in techniques invented by physicians to change the course of illness, and in judgments by them as to when to leave well enough alone and allow nature to take its course. An ability to balance artificial and natural forces, and to weigh in the decision technical, ethical, and social factors, was the essence of Hippocratic thinking on the matter. The perspective is stated boldly in this passage from *The Art*: "If a man demands from an art a power over what does not belong to the art, or from nature a power that does not belong to nature, his ignorance is more allied to madness than to lack of knowledge. For in cases where we may have the mastery through the means afforded by a natural constitution or by an art, there we may be craftsmen but nowhere else. Whenever therefore a man suffers from an ill which is too strong for the means at the disposal of medicine, he surely must not even expect that it can be overcome by medicine."[28]

The passage sends a message of caution to those seeking to draw from therapy a power it does not have. It labels such action as flawed medical thinking and urges physicians to limit interventions to those cases in which they stand a chance of benefiting patients. Hippocratic physicians were concerned with limiting the harm of therapy to patients and retaining public confidence in the judgment of doctors and the learning of medicine. The Hippocratics viewed actions in which doctors exceeded the limits of their craft as hubris. For medical arrogance not only endangered the reputation of the involved doctor but by extension threatened public confidence in medicine itself.

Pius XII expressed a remarkably parallel concern when he endeavored to place limits on the use of the artificial respirator. Like the Hippocratics, he warned of a threat posed by therapy that extended beyond its physical harm to the patient. His concern was that the critical focus on spiritual ends when illness afflicted human life could be tellingly diverted by fruitless efforts to salvage the body. Though separated by two and a half millennia and vastly different thinking, the Hippocratic and Catholic traditions identified factors external to therapy as critical limiting guides to its use.

The story of artificial respiration is a tale of expansiveness meeting limit. That is the essence of the Quinlan case. Repeatedly in the legal decision about it, the court justifies the legitimacy of its intervention into medical care. It asserts that community values must coexist with medical ones in decisions on patient care and sets in motion a process to achieve a sociomedical consensus through a multidisciplinary ethics committee. In the years that have passed since the Quinlan case, social innovations have appeared in parallel with technological advances, which endeavored to place limits on their use. These innovations fall roughly into three categories: those initiated by governments, physicians, and medical institutions.

Government-sponsored limits were introduced in 1976, the same year as the Quinlan decision, when California became the first state to pass a natural death act. The act gave adults the legal right to control decisions respecting their medical care, including the right to have life-supporting technologies withheld or withdrawn in the presence of a terminal condition. The bill gave standing to the significance of "patient dignity," whose loss, along with the pain and suffering of the illness, was to be weighed against the value of therapy. It created a procedure through which the patient's views could be expressed in the form of a written directive to the physician. The directive could be revoked at any time by patients and gave physicians who acted on it relief from civil liability.[29] It became known popularly as a living will. By the 1990s legislation to validate living wills had been adopted throughout the country. At this time an allied patient-focused innovation through which the use of technology could be limited appeared, the durable power of attorney for health care. It enabled individuals to designate a person to make decisions on their behalf when they were incapacitated and unable to provide guidance about their own care.

Physician-centered limits have been focused on clinical orders that prevent the initiation of technological procedures. The first, whose use began in the mid-1970s was the do-not-resuscitate (DNR) order. It was designed to deter invasive efforts to resuscitate patients who were terminally ill and suffered a circulatory or respiratory catastrophe that would kill them. A joint and documented agreement by doctor and patient not to call for emergency cardiopulmonary resuscitation (CPR), if such an event occurred, was placed in the patient's record as a DNR order. Thus, the DNR order was a response to the growing use of CPR.

But at the Hermann Hospital in Houston in the late 1980s a wider approach to meet the needs of such patients was implemented through a document the author helped develop called a supportive care protocol. One of the reasons that patients who were imminently dying received technological interventions that had the basic result of prolonging their suffering, was the absence of a therapeutic viewpoint focused on moderating suffering rather than prolonging life. The supportive care protocol provided this to hospital staff and the patients they served. Its innovative feature was extending the concept behind withholding CPR to a range of other therapies such as antibiotics or kidney dialysis whose use, like CPR, were judged by doctors and terminally ill patients to prolong the dying process rather than to provide medical benefit: further, these therapies could be not only withheld but also discontinued. In addition, the protocol suggested measures to add to the care of these patients such as increased interventions by social workers and chaplains. While the tradition of hospice is to treat terminally ill patients in a spirit of relieving suffering, this attitude is difficult to establish in hospitals geared as they are to technological intervention directed at life preservation. The supportive care protocol not only proposed therapy but also carried a message: purpose, determined jointly by doctor and patient (or surrogate decision-maker), should control the use of technology.

Institution-based limits on technology have centered on the creation of ethics committees, which the 1976 Quinlan case catapulted to national attention.[30] Within a decade, the committee was entrenched in American hospitals connected to academic institutions, which provided them with members trained in ethics. Now, it is a common feature of American hospital life. Its main function has been what it was in the Quinlan case: to adjudicate the problems of maintaining or withdrawing life support. These committees have evolved to incorporate as members not only physicians, lawyers, and clergy but also nurses, administrative staff, and community representatives, and they largely see their opinions on cases as advisory, not binding. Wisely, they recognize that their view of cases is restricted, and that clinicians and families have not only greater knowledge about a case involving them but specific legal and ethical obligations in making choices. Many committees seek to educate hospital staff about ethical issues and help the hospital rewrite rules and procedures that bear on ethical matters. Most committees do not seek to extend their reach beyond life-threatening cases, which has limited their potential to develop a comprehensive ethical awareness in hospital staff.

At times, the intervention of an ethics committee fails to resolve the conflicts about end-of-life care. Given a standstill on how to proceed in a case when physicians and families and patients are on different sides, and cases when the patient, for medical or economic reasons, cannot leave for another hospital, the traditional route taken is to the courthouse, as in the Quinlan episode. In the mid-1980s articles began to appear in the medical literature on what was called futile treatment. It was defined as a conclusion, based on personal experience or scientific data, that further lifesaving treatment of a particular patient who was dying was futile. Reaching such a conclusion, the argument went, relieved the physician of an ethical obligation to continue such care. In 1999 Texas passed a law that legally sanctioned the creation of a special ethics consultation committee to resolve such disputes between families and doctors. If the committee failed in this effort but found the case futile, the hospital was empowered to transfer the patient to another treatment facility. If after ten days this proved impossible, the hospital and the physicians could lawfully withhold or withdraw the treatments that were futile, even over the objections of the patient or family.[31] Questions arise as to whether the futility predictions of the committees have scientific validity, whether such a process is preferable to traditional resort to the courts, and whether the existence of such a committee short-circuits dialogue between the parties as the ultimate means to resolve conflict.[32] Thus, the discourse continues.

In the tale "the Sorcerer's Apprentice," the apprentice unleashes the power of the sorcerer and cannot restore the order of things. The story of the artificial respirator has features of this tale. To practice modern medicine is often to feel overwhelmed by its technology. The artificial respirator not only works automatically but often seems to gain an independence of action once it is unleashed by the hand of the doctor writing the order for it. This is an inherent property of technologies designed to be self-governing. Yet the ability to change therapeutic direction in step with a change in patient condition is the essence not only of scientific care but also of ethical practice, and a crucial role for ethics in such matters is to provide the force of moral argument to challenge the automaticity of the machine.

5

THE QUEST TO UNIFY
HEALTH CARE THROUGH
THE PATIENT RECORD

The breadth of American health care is enormous. It involves thousands of health institutions and millions of health professionals, who each year treat hundreds of millions of patients with billions of tests and therapies. The information generated about this mass of people and the therapies they receive must be brought together somewhere, to integrate the medical biography and technological evaluations of their illnesses and to provide critical data for the administrative management, insurance reimbursement, educational study, and scientific investigation of care. That *somewhere* is the patient record. This multipage paper tome or its computer-based counterpart is a crucial technology because of its unique role in binding together the enterprise of health care. How well has the patient record achieved its mission, and what are its future prospects?

Early efforts to build a sound patient record in America were auspicious. In 1821 the Massachusetts General Hospital (MGH), one of the first and most effective hospitals in the United States, opened in Boston. At its founding, trustees and staff decided to systematically record the evidence generated by the care of patients. James Jackson, a founder and leading doctor at MGH, described in 1836 how records were produced about the some three hundred patients the hospital treated each year:

On the entrance of a patient, the house physician (usually a medical pupil in his third year, and always a resident in the hospital), collects and writes down the history of the case and the actual state of the patient. The physician visits the hospital every morning, and examines every patient daily. He dictates aloud the record of the day at the bedside of each patient, and the prescriptions, if there be any. All this is recorded at the moment by the house physician, in a first book, or journal, where the record goes on continuously from one patient to another. Before the visit of the following day, the record thus made is transferred to a case-book, under the head of each case; a process similar to that of posting from a mercantile journal into a ledger. This case-book is carried round by the physician in his daily visits; and, as he arrives at the bedside of each patient, he opens to his case. At this time there are sixty-eight case-books filled in this manner.[1]

A study I made of nineteenth-century MGH records found that those from the 1820s and 1830s contained sparse details about the patient's history, family, or social activities. They start with a note on age and occupation, followed by an account of how the illness developed, findings of physical examination, and reports of daily progress. The 1840s records are much the same but devote more space to the patient's previous illnesses. By the 1870s graphs appeared that separately summarize the daily numeric entries of pulse rate, respiratory rate, and temperature. The graphic method of depiction gave doctors an immediate sense of either stability or change in the vital functions. Additions made during the 1880s and 1890s include a chart that tracked chemical analyses of the urine, stamped outlines of the abdomen and chest to denote the location of physical signs of illness, and the notation of findings from blood and bacteriologic studies.[2]

The records reflect the development of nineteenth-century medicine. Early in the century, physicians extended their senses into the interior of the body through simple instruments like the stethoscope and ophthalmoscope. By its second half, much attention was given to evaluating the physiological and chemical state of the body and to depicting the findings using graphs and numbers.[3] Many doctors believed such data were more dependable than either the patient's experiences or the physician's sensory observations made with instruments like the stethoscope. These types of evidence were lumped together as tainted by a subjective essence difficult for others to confirm and dependent on imprecise verbal statements to convey meaning. Numerically based and graphic data seemed free of these deficiencies and to have an accuracy appropriate to scientific medicine. Such evidence became highly significant to the record's development and was increasingly displayed in the patient record as the nineteenth century came to a close.

But most records written in that period in the United States were not kept as carefully as those at MGH and reflected neither the progress made in medicine nor the care given to patients. Many doctors believed a careful, handwritten narrative of the procedures of examination, diagnostic findings, therapy, or results of care was unnecessary. They thought of the record as a private document owned by them whose purpose was to trigger the recall of observations made and therapies given to patients, the principal gist of which they carried about in their heads. Lacking pressure from outside sources such as professional, social, or legal institutions for an accounting of practice results, the record's form, content, and use could be and was determined by each doctor personally. Thus, the medical literature of the nineteenth century contains few remarks on routine keeping of clinical records by doctors, and even when given, the comments usually are dropped into discussions of other issues. For example, in the midst of comments on auscultation a physician writing in 1861 urged his colleagues "to take notes not of your diagnosis, but of the *grounds on which you base it*. It is of no use to yourself, your patient, or to science to remember that on such a day, you thought that there was pneumonia or tubercle, but it is of great use to all to remember why you thought so."[4]

Most hospitals were little better than private practitioners at record keeping. Writing of European hospitals in the mid-nineteenth century, the founder of modern nursing, Florence Nightingale, tells us: "There is a growing conviction that in all hospitals, even those which are best conducted, there is a great and unnecessary waste of life.... In attempting to arrive at the truth, I have applied everywhere for information, but in scarcely an instance have I been able to obtain hospital records fit for any purposes of comparison."[5]

In the United States it was much the same. For example, clinicians associated with an innovative practice begun in the late nineteenth century, formed under the aegis of the Mayo brothers at the St. Mary's Hospital in Rochester, Minnesota, produced early records sorely deficient in detail about clinical findings. In ones written between 1885 and 1907, the diagnosis and therapy given are omitted about half the time. Indeed, it can be difficult to learn from these records whether a patient had surgery. In some cases, this has to be inferred from notes found in the margin of the record, such as "died six months after operation." All that many of the records contain are the patient's name, admission date, age, residence, and brief statements of the presenting complaint, such as "gas on the stomach and poor sleep."[6] Thus, in the nineteenth century the patient record was not regarded by most practitioners and hospitals as an important aspect of practice.

In the early twentieth century, the record underwent great scrutiny in the United States as the data it held became important in three significant areas: the reform of American medical education, the rise of concern about the quality of care in hospitals, and the growth of a technology-driven specialization of practice.

As the new century began, records were singled out as central devices for changing the instruction of medical students and hospital staff. At the vanguard of this effort was Walter Cannon, a student at Harvard Medical School who later achieved fame there as a physiologist. Cannon was troubled by three features of his education: an excessive reliance on the lecture to transmit knowledge, an inability to follow patients over time to view the development of their illness, and the difficulty of seeing an adequate number of patients who exhibited the typical disorders students would encounter in practice. His solution, published in a 1900 paper, used the records of patients as the keys to learning medicine. This strategy replaced the passive instruction of lectures with real-life situations portrayed in records of doctors and patients meeting illness. He was fortunate to have close at hand Harvard faculty and teaching hospitals such as MGH, where detailed patient records were kept and available. Wrote Cannon: "Cases of all the types, variations and complications of almost every disease are to be found in hospital records or in records of the private practice of instructors. These records include a history of family tendencies, notes of previous illness, an account of the onset of the attack, the results of physical examination at the hospital, the story of the ups and downs in the course of the disease, the treatment with its modifications as the symptoms changed, and, in case of death, possibly the findings of autopsy."[7] Cannon drew his idea from the work of Professor C. C. Langdell of Harvard Law School, who thirty years earlier had introduced the case method of instruction into legal education. For its use in teaching medicine, essential data from the chart were abstracted and presented to students, who then attempted to provide a diagnosis, suggest appropriate therapy, and indicate the likely outcome of care.

The patient's record became the center of a basic change in the education of the house staff and attending physicians in hospitals when in 1910 Richard C. Cabot, a physician at MGH, and James Homer Wright, a pathologist there, began to hold weekly exercises together. In them, Cabot discussed with the hospital staff the clinical evidence and reasoning leading to the diagnosis of a presented case, and Wright provided autopsy evidence that confirmed or opposed the clinical diagnosis. The origin of these clinical-pathological conferences (as they were called) was the result of an abiding interest that Cabot displayed throughout his medical life: learning from mistakes. This stemmed from an incident in 1908 when, looking through hospital records at MGH, he discovered that a particular case had been diagnosed as neurasthenia and an autopsy performed. Yet in the autopsy records, kept separately in the pathology laboratory, it stated that the patient had died of cancer. "What especially impressed me," he wrote, "was that the clinical diagnosis had never been changed, presumably because the clinicians had been unaware of the post-mortem result."[8] This led to his initiative to hold the weekly conferences.

Medical observers were enthralled by the dynamics of these meetings. Wrote one: "It is skill and scholarship pitted against the unknown. For the moment the dingy pathological amphitheater becomes a jousting field. At the end of the discussion there is a moment of tense suspense while the pathologist, not without a sense of the dramatic value of the situation, comes forward to herald the outcome of the encounter. Defeated or in laurels, the clinician goes his way – in either case a better diagnostician."[9] While the concept of correlating clinical findings and autopsy reports was at the heart of the nineteenth-century movement that had introduced physical diagnosis into medicine, the idea of using medical records to teach about the correlations was new. Cabot continually stressed that the objective of the discussions was not just to determine the correct diagnosis. More significant were the lessons taught in analyzing data, weighing alternatives, and determining the connections between clinical findings and autopsy evidence. The exercises were so successful in enlightening even accomplished clinicians that the hospital began in 1915 to publish them by subscription as "Case Records of the Massachusetts General Hospital." In 1923, these discussions of patient records reached an even larger audience when they were published regularly in the forerunner of the *New England Journal of Medicine*, in which they continue to be featured.[10]

Just as educators regarded the patient record with new eyes, so too did physicians who were concerned with the quality of care. At the forefront of this movement was the American College of Surgeons (ACS), a professional organization committed to bettering surgical practice. The record assumed importance shortly after ACS was founded in 1913, when it decided to base admission on a review of one hundred records of operations submitted by candidates. To the dismay of reviewers, the data in the records received were sketchy, ordered in different forms, and lacking in detail concerning procedure and purpose. As a result, ACS decided to make reform of the patient record a priority, as it now focused on the need for raising standards in medical care. The first object in its view was the hospital.

The growth of American hospitals had been spectacular in the previous four decades, fueled by technologic innovations that made them safer and more effective. Numbering about four hundred in 1875, there were more than four thousand hospitals by 1909, and almost seven thousand by 1917. To secure the societal confidence and support necessary for hospitals to flourish, ACS decided that publicly announced standards of the care given in them were needed. It collected data on patient care from questionnaires sent to hospitals in the United States and Canada, and conferred with many physicians and administrators. From these activities, it developed and announced in 1918 standards to discriminate good from poor hospitals. Judgments were based on the existence of effective procedures to govern the conduct of the hospital staff and to determine the qualifications of doctors seeking to admit and treat patients, the adequacy of radiological and laboratory facilities, and the state of patient records. To meet the standard for records, hospitals were required to keep them on all patients, with each record containing a summary of clinically significant events. Hospitals further were to use the records to analyze the outcomes of medical and surgical procedures, with a view to prevent future error. Here, ACS entered new territory, the road to which had been paved by a bold and controversial orthopedic surgeon at MGH, Ernest Amory Codman.

Codman was born in Boston in 1869, attended Harvard College, and graduated from Harvard Medical School in 1895. An avid hunter of grouse, he kept a precise account of the ratio of shells used to birds shot, an index of his efficiency as a marksman. It was a harbinger of what would become the focus of his medical life – determining the factors that led to successful or unsuccessful outcomes of care (Figure 11). His first opportunity to assert this interest was as a medical student administering anesthesia to surgical patients at MGH. He and a fellow student, Harvey Cushing, who would become America's pioneering brain surgeon, vied for the best patient outcomes, with the winner buying the loser dinner at the end of his anesthesia rotation (who paid is unclear). Codman wrote a paper about his experience but never published it because the faculty thought his comments on the cases who died were too frank for the good of the hospital.

In 1900 Codman became an assistant surgeon at MGH and began examining the outcomes of care on the surgical service in which he worked. Despite the fact that MGH kept what were undoubtedly the most precise records of each patient's care in this period, the outcomes of their care, published each year in the hospital's annual report, were stated only in broad categories, such as whether they were well at discharge or had their symptoms partly relieved or unrelieved. Codman determined to learn the state of discharged patients a year after treatment by inducing them to return to the hospital for reexamination. This would be a far better index of the success or failure of their treatment than brief discharge comments in the record. The chief of Codman's surgical service, pleased with his work, had the findings entered into the patient records. From then on, Codman devoted himself to exploring the relation between treatments and their outcomes, and the consequences of this knowledge for all involved with the case.[11]

As ACS engaged in discussions of hospital standards, Codman, who had been chosen as the first chair of its standards committee, presented to the organization what he called his end-result system. He created the system to deal with the failure of physicians to be accountable for the results of their therapies to patients, colleagues, hospital overseers, and the public. Without a clear view of the end results of therapy, patients chose doctors and doctors themselves often evaluated colleagues on the basis of the vagaries of reputation and personality. Codman wanted hospitals to assess systematically the factors determining the therapeutic

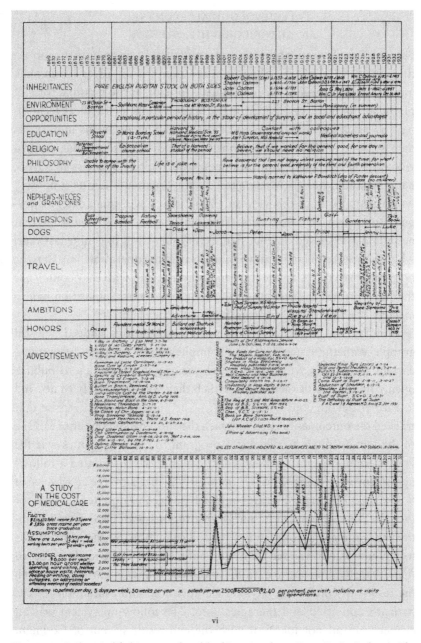

Figure 11. Codman's life history, reduced by him to a chart. From E. A. Codman. *The Shoulder*...Boston: 1934, vi. Reprinted by Krieger Publishing, Malabar, Fla., 1984, and used with permission of the publisher. This illustration demonstrates his mastery of compressing and arraying data in a form that generates synthesis and understanding of them. In this case, it shows how Codman became who he was and reveals the honest and incisive intellectual perspective that drove his pioneering work in studying the end results (now referred to as outcomes) of medical care and making the case for making them public.

outcome of each patient through accumulating basic data on diagnoses, therapy, and the results of care. In the event of an adverse outcome, inquiry into its origins was necessary – looking at the possible roles of physician, patient, disease, hospital organization, or medical technology. The patient record was to be the crucial agent in this inquiry, its data serving to determine responsibility and, with this done, to provide evidence to guide future choices to accrediting agencies like ACS, patients, and others.[12] Many agreed with Codman. "Let us suppose," wrote a supporter of this view in 1919, "that a workman enters a hospital and learns he needs an operation for hernia. It is reasonable that he should ask: 'Based on your figures for other cases like mine last year, what chances have I to be at work again after the operation?'. . . Can the hospital answer it? Can the staff and officers claim with easy conscience that they protect the welfare of this man by every safeguard known to medical science? If so, how can they prove the claim?"[13]

Codman was ahead of his time in his suggestions (indeed, we still grapple with the issues he posed). Implementation of his recommendations required a willingness by physicians and hospitals to publish openly the results of their work, which they were not ready to do, and to further devote considerable energy and funds to an enterprise that tracked the outcomes of care, at which they also balked (Figure 12). One of the few hospitals to develop a program to track outcomes was the Presbyterian Hospital in New York, which in 1914 initiated a follow-up system in surgery. This action was influenced by the new view of hospitals as no longer charities in which physicians donated services for the care of the poor but as public institutions with clear responsibilities that required accountability for clinical action. At the heart of this follow-up system was the follow-up note, a part of the medical record that detailed admitting symptoms and those found at subsequent visits, the results of continuing physical examination, and evaluations of the patient's condition and therapies used. The follow-up system was an element of and not identical with the end-result system of Codman. The latter not only required the following of cases to determine the outcome of the treatment but also demanded analysis of the causes of the outcome and the application of this knowledge to avoid future errors and encourage future successes.[14]

While in this period the end-result and follow-up systems were not widely adopted, ACS convinced many hospitals to hold monthly staff

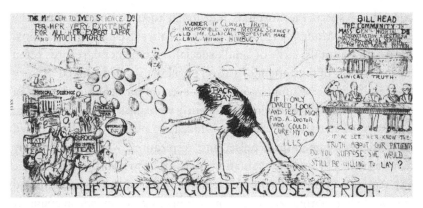

Figure 12. The Back Bay, Golden Goose–Ostrich cartoon. From Codman EA, *The Shoulder*...Boston: 1934, xxvi. Reprinted by Krieger Publishing Co., Malabar, Fla., 1984 and used with permission of the publisher. Codman's efforts to implement his end-result idea in Boston met resistance, which he attributed largely to the medical community's concern that public disclosure of practice outcomes might diminish their income. In response, he sponsored a forum in 1916 at the Boston Medical Library to discuss hospital efficiency and patient outcomes. However, under a cover behind the stage, Codman had secretly prepared an eight-foot-long cartoon ready for display at the end of the program to use if, as he assumed, no presenter or audience member raised the role of money in the end-result debate. Codman described the cartoon as follows:

It depicts President Lowell [of Harvard] standing on the Cambridge Bridge, wondering whether it would be possible for the professors of the Medical School to support themselves on their salaries, if they had no opportunity to practice among the rich people of the Back Bay [of Boston]. The Back Bay is represented as an ostrich with her head in a pile of sand, devouring humbugs and kicking out her golden eggs blindly to the professors, who show more interest in the golden eggs than they do in Medical Science. On the right is the Massachusetts General Hospital with its board of trustees deliberating as to whether, if they really used the End Result System, and let the Back Bay know how many mistakes were made on the hospital patients, they would still be willing to give her golden eggs to support the hospital, and would still employ the members of their staff and thus save the expense of salaries. Across the river and over the hill are seen armies of medical students coming to Harvard because they have heard that the End Result System will be installed in her affiliated hospitals.[1]

When the cartoon was unveiled at the forum's end, astonishment spread through the audience. Some walked out in protest; others were amused; a few congratulated Codman. "For some months," he wrote, "I was in disgrace, but the publicity obtained, which spread not only in our local papers but in those of all the other large cities, fulfilled my expectations."[2] So his views on end results received the important public discussion he had desired.

References: 1. Ibid., xxvii–viii.
2. Ibid., xxv.

meetings at which therapeutic outcomes were discussed and to begin to document the actions they took more systematically, which entailed focusing attention on the patient record for evidence of what happened.

In this respect, the hospitals had much to overcome. In 1917 the editor of the *Modern Hospital*, John Hornby, declared that in most American hospitals, large or small, specialized or general, records often lacked reports of the patient's history, physical examination, laboratory test results, or a presumptive diagnosis even on those about to have an operation. Daily progress notes frequently were missing, too. He found, generally, that only the charts produced by nurses, which recorded the patients' temperature, pulse, and respiration, were appropriately maintained.[15] In its first evaluation in 1918, in which the state of the 617 American hospitals with more than a hundred beds was examined and publicly reported, ACS confirmed Hornby's pessimistic account. It found that fewer than half had adequate records.[16]

Several factors accounted for the shoddy condition of records. Like their nineteenth-century predecessors, many doctors in the post–First World War period continued to think of records as memory aids, with the bulk of the patient data kept in their heads. Physicians also were afraid that the growing modern call to place data on their patients in hospital records, out of their control, endangered the confidential nature of medical communications. Many doctors opposed to this claimed that they kept good records on patients in their offices, thereby protecting confidentiality and having at hand the data they needed.

However, separate studies by Allen Peebles[17] and by Osler Peterson[18] revealed the sad truth of the private office record in the first half of the twentieth century: there was little data in it to be guided by or confidential about. Less than a fifth of the doctors studied kept complete records containing basic evidence on history, diagnosis, and therapy. Some kept no records, and the majority of accounts were fragmentary. The most common cause of such poor records was the pressure of practice on available time; retaining facts in the memory was more time conserving than a written documentation of actions. But Peterson showed how greatly flawed even the remembered account of illness was, and thus how unjustified the notion that detailed written records were not necessary. He found that the typical physician who practiced in a small town might know much about the personal lives of patients – who their relatives were and what school they attended – but could not summon up critical facts about the medical lives of their patients. For example, when asked about a surgical scar on one of his patients, a physician remembered sending the patient to a medical center for care but could recall neither the nature of the illness nor the type of surgery used to treat it. "To expect a physician to remember," wrote Peterson, "all or even most of the facts about three or four thousand patients whom he has seen a variable number of times in the preceding year or two is to expect prodigies of memory beyond human capacity. When he sees patients at the rate of 25 to 50 a day, all pertinent details simply cannot be retained."

Physicians were not alone in thwarting efforts for good record keeping. Joining them were many hospitals, which balked at allocating funds for the dictation machines, stenographers, and librarians needed to transcribe, store, and retrieve patient records. A typical consequence of this neglect occurred in a Philadelphia hospital, which lost 285 records in one year. This, ACS reported in 1924, was mainly due to poor record management.[19] However, changes in the technology and practice of medicine provided additional ammunition to overcome doctor and hospital resistance to adequately documenting their care of patients.

Physicians in the early twentieth century had begun to face new challenges to their ability to absorb an expanding body of medical knowledge and the technology that accompanied it. One response was to narrow the scope of practice and specialize in a given area. Specialization was not new to medicine, but the pressures to embrace it were greater in this period than in any previous one.

The growth of the hospital itself was in part a response to specialization. It brought together generalists and specialists in a single geographic locus, facilitating expeditious consultation and the sharing of judgments among them. In addition to physicians, a growing cadre of nurses and other newly created personnel such as medical social workers required a spatial proximity to one another to compare their distinctive knowledge. However, the separate observations made by this increasingly diverse hospital staff would fail to provide their full benefit to the patient if what transpired was not preserved for others on the staff to see.

Written records that accurately reflected interventions thus were essential to the new level of coordination demanded by a fragmenting medicine. The record written in an abbreviated language as a reminder to the doctor or stored in the doctor's memory, although fraught with the dangers of forgetting or conflating observations, nonetheless was conceivable in an age when medicine was the domain of the individual. But in the organized cooperative system that medicine was becoming, written disclosure and clear depiction of findings was essential. Still, convincing doctors to respond to the new situation was not easy. Wrote an observer in 1924: "The mistake that we made in former times was to leave the recording of cases to the pleasure and convenience of the surgeon. Usually he never found it convenient – under the old regime we looked to the individual and not to the organization."[20] Two pivotal innovations in this period encouraged doctors to coordinate medical care through the record. One was the concept of a record-keeping system that unified the patient's hospital visits; the other aimed to standardize the collection and notation of medical data.

Even in those hospitals that kept good records in the nineteenth century, data on any given patient were scattered. For example, at MGH, separate sets of records bound in volumes were kept by the medical and surgical services, but even the therapeutic interventions made on a patient in a single hospital visit to one of the departments might be noted on widely separated pages in a particular volume. While references were given to pages where the patient's record was continued and index volumes of admitted patients were constructed on the medical and surgical services, no similar system was created at MGH to handle records of outpatient visits, which were not even bound in volumes but stored in drawers and separate from medical and surgical service records. Thus, even at a hospital committed to good record keeping, as MGH was, it was difficult for any clinician to construct a total picture of the patient's care.

An effort to bring together in a single place all the medical visits of a patient occurred first at the St. Mary's Hospital overseen by the Mayo brothers in 1907. But such a unified record was extensively developed at the Presbyterian Hospital in New York City, which in 1916 had created a single locus containing the data on all interventions a patient received at the hospital.[21] Its goal was no less than keeping a "life history of an individual in one cover."[22] Advocates of the need for such efficient records bolstered their arguments by emphasizing the hospital's corporate nature. If no bank or other significant business of this period would tolerate an ineffective record system, why, asked reformers, should the hospital? The unit concept, as it was called, greatly increased the efficiency of using the record, although its adoption was impeded by, among other things, the additional personnel and expense required to manage it, and delays in a central system of data storage created to gain rapid clinical access to its data.

Having the discontinuous treatment patients received over the course of an illness or a life unified in a single space through the record assisted the coordination necessary in the evolving system of specialized medical care. However, more effective integration of these data was only part of the problem. Of what use was the more efficient collation in the record of data for research or patient care if the data were flawed? A central figure in the movement to standardize clinical data was Raymond Pearl, chief statistician at the Johns Hopkins Hospital and professor of vital statistics at the university's School of Public Health.

Pearl's key objective in his 1920s work was to create a scientific clinical record in which quantitative expression reigned. He lauded the trend in medicine, begun in the second half of the nineteenth century, to seek quantitative measures of illness. By the early twentieth century, this interest had resulted in a growth in laboratory procedures and the increasing use of graphic evidence produced by devices such as the electrocardiograph. But the statistical treatment of evidence had progressed more slowly than appreciation or collection of the evidence itself. While it was true that hospitals routinely published work statistics (e.g., admission rates, diseases treated, patients discharged alive or dead), these figures often were collected more to show donors that the hospital had met its moral responsibilities than to advance medical knowledge.

Pearl argued that medicine could become an exact science if it used quantitative methods to statistically capture the enormous number of facts (both subjective and objective) that the treatment of patients generated. He envisioned turning the patient record, filled with such data, into an engine for scientific advance. But this required hospitals to have a statistical department to assemble, classify, index, and analyze data. Recognizing the labor this required, he recommended the transfer of selected items of information from case histories onto punched cards, which could be analyzed by mechanical tabulation machines newly invented by Herman Hollerith.

But problems clouded Pearl's vision of such knowledge creation. The trustees of many large hospitals of the 1920s did not focus on the infrastructure of record librarians, stenographers, and statisticians needed to enhance the clinical and scientific value of the patient record. They basically did not understand the value of such records or the analysis of their contents, and hence the need to expend much resources on them. The same was true at small hospitals. They were thought to need at least a record librarian to facilitate the entry of medical procedures promptly and to be sure that basic data such as history, physical examination, and diagnosis were transcribed and progress notes made. But support for even this modest step was poor.

As to the evidence in the record itself, the most glaring flaw was the omission of important facts about patients, such as their sex, weight, age, or social circumstances. The chief cause of this flaw was variability of content and organization by the individual doctors who wrote the record. Pearl noted, in perhaps the first statement of the garbage in, garbage out principle of data collection: "Since one cannot get out of any machinery of statistical treatment anything intrinsically different from what went in, it follows that accuracy and completeness of the initial routine statistical data collected in the hospital are matters of prime importance."[23] Pearl's solution was a standard history form to cover the basic facts of all diseases and special ones for frequently found disorders. He realized that no general form sufficed to contain all the pertinent facts of the patient's history: hence, he thought physicians should be free to write what they wished in another section of the record. Still, he knew the proposal would stir opposition: "One realizes," he wrote in 1921,

that any suggestion in the direction of standardizing case writing by the process of putting into operation methods which have been found sound and useful in other branches of science and in modern business, will at once be scornfully or even derisively received by some. It will be argued that any such process tends to cramp their individuality. This argument is perfectly valid. It will inordinately cramp such portion of their individuality as finds its expression in carelessness, inaccuracy, forgetfulness, and inattentive observation. Insofar as it is desirable to foster and preserve these intellectual qualities, and embalm their results in the permanent archives of a hospital, clinicians and surgeons should be encouraged to go on writing histories in the old way.[24]

Still, doctors were concerned that the gains of uniformity would be offset by the loss of what made a patient's illness unique. Thus, they persisted in writing records that displayed a personal stamp.

After the Second World War, medical research and technological advances grew exponentially, heightening the burden on the medical record, already overstressed by the volume of information within its covers. While Pearl's messages about the record went largely unheard as the new century had progressed, nonetheless, they were vital. For the increase in technological procedures conducted beyond the bedside in cubicles scattered about the hospital – such as laboratory analysis and radiological imaging – caused a torrent of reports to flow into the chart on separate slips. Complementing them were notes written by consultants, whose numbers grew as specialization began to take hold of medicine.

The result, as I found in the archives of MGH, was a record made into a scrapbook. In the 1910s and 1920s, technological findings and consultants' comments frequently were pasted on the margins of records, often obscuring clinical observations and progress notes. Putting together the clinical sequence and logic of these multiple observations was difficult and even perilous, for as the pages of the record were turned, one faced the possibility that the paste holding the reports might not hold and their original site of residence be forever lost; thus, using them required considerable caution.[25] By the 1940s and 1950s, hundred-page documents were not uncommon, at MGH and elsewhere, weighing down not only the arms but also the minds of clinicians who sought to extract from them the story of their patients' illness. As this became increasingly difficult, many physicians started from scratch when they met patients anew. Thus, the patient's history of illness was asked for repeatedly. And with each recounting, time invariably caused details of the story to change, making it difficult for the doctor to know which was the most authentic version. Laboratory tests also were repeated since previous studies were not easily found in the record. Even when discursive material such as histories of illness or consultants' notes were located, they were sometimes illegible or fragmentary, thus creating another rationale for duplicated efforts.

The dispersion of the patient's medical data also caused problems. The irony was not lost on physicians of having in hand an already-voluminous patient record, and recognizing it was but one chapter of a story, spread among not only other services within the hospital but also record rooms of other hospitals and doctors' office files, not only in the same but in other towns and cities. If this were not enough, the volume of data overflowing the covers of medical records was matched by that coming off medical presses to dwell between the covers of journals and books. Wherever doctors turned, they were met by more information than they could meaningfully assimilate. So when stories began to appear at the start of the 1960s of how a properly programmed computer was able to gather, integrate, analyze, store, and retrieve prodigious quantities of medical information with ease, doctors' interest immediately was piqued.

But by the end of the 1960s, a decade after clinicians had begun to apply the computer to clinical work, the expectation that it would rescue them from the straits of the information explosion had not been borne out. This failure had many causes: anxiety by physician users that computers might challenge their authority; difficulty in mastering computer terminology and operation; a coincident increase rather than decrease compared to paper records in the time spent entering data into the record; the high cost of bringing computers to hospitals and physicians' offices; an inability to define adequately the logic used by physicians to reach decisions and to mimic it in computer programs focused on diagnosis; the difficulty of reeducating staff to learn a new technology in which they feared they might never be expert; the ineffectiveness of computers in improving collegial communication, a result of the lack of systemwide adoption of the technology; and a view that the cost and time of learning a new computerized information system was not worth the effort and gains. As one observer put it:

By the mid-1960's vendors were selling "packages" for the automation of hospital functions; vendor marketing advertisements were translated into awesome promises. The computer was hailed as an eventual replacement for the physician, an efficient manager of medical records, and an instrument which would soon eliminate the human element in data acquisition, processing, and interpretation.... Many hospitals acquired computers and attempted to implement complex computer-based information systems with acquisition, communication and processing features. For many, the experience was costly and counter-productive. Hospital administrators, laboratory directors and others responsible for system acquisition quickly discovered limitations in the technology, and the difficulty of bringing systems to an operational state became apparent.[26]

A basic problem in the diffusion of the computer in clinical medicine was excessive expectations for it. The computer was presented to clinicians in the early 1960s as a superbrain that would solve in short order the data problem of medicine through its ability to hold and retrieve information, the diagnosis problem of medicine through its ability to transform large quantities of evidence into disease patterns, and the workload problem of medicine through programs that allowed patients to interact directly with computers to diagnose and even to treat disease, as programs that facilitated psychotherapy attempted to demonstrate as feasible. But these goals were unrealistic.

Supporters of this innovation largely directed their attention to the computer's internal capabilities, focusing essentially on its technical characteristics rather than judging its use and measuring expectations for it according to its fit with the surrounding clinical and social environments. The basic mistake they made, and one often seen with medical innovations, was not to view the computer as a technology embedded in a set of complicated associations: with other technologies, with a system of values that directed the user's actions, with financial systems, and so forth. The dovetailing of an invention with impinging technical and social systems, particularly one with the unique characteristics of a computer, takes time. Gradually, this was recognized. Further, the problems of developing programs to mimic the clinical logic used by physicians (as was tried first) or developing new patterns of logic not used in human thought (as was attempted later) were found by investigators to be much more complicated than they anticipated and to require long periods of study and trial before the results wanted could be achieved.

Doctors in the 1960s also were concerned about language and vocabulary problems associated with computer use. The different languages used by the engineers and physical scientists who designed computers and developed programs for them, and by the physicians who would use the results, proved significant barriers to cooperation between them and slowed program development. Further, while the computer might help standardize the formats through which data were arrayed, there was inadequate recognition of the barriers ahead to developing a standard vocabulary to go along with a regularized and legible format. In pioneering work, Alvan Feinstein and his colleagues at Yale in the 1960s demonstrated that the main source of variability among physicians observing a given clinical phenomenon was not differences in perception or what they saw or heard. Rather, it was the criteria and vocabulary used to describe the perceived event. It was only when the Feinstein group specified criteria and vocabulary to identify a clinical sign that diagnostic disagreements among them began to recede.[27] The problem of developing and implementing a standardized language of discourse for use in computerized patient records based on a common view of clinical description, such as Feinstein advocated, remains unresolved.

Predictions were more restrained in the 1970s about how quickly the computer could achieve the necessary technological capabilities to assist in medical data handling and decision making, as well as overcome psychological, social, and economic barriers to its acceptance and use. Significant advances, however, were made in specialized areas of medical diagnosis. Computer programs to detect disorders, such as one for rheumatic heart disease, were able to best clinicians in a diagnostic competition. Graphic data such as the tracings of electrocardiographs or pictorial data such as the images of X-rays were being converted into numeric formats that facilitated their analysis by computers.

Some of the most interesting work of this period on computers and the record came from the physician Lawrence Weed. He reorganized the format of the patient record by directing the focus of clinicians to the physical dysfunctions and social issues necessary to treat in meeting a patient's illness rather than to the usual ordering of data according to the source from which it came (e.g., doctor, nurse, laboratory) or to the traditional diagnostic categories that named the diseases from which the patient suffered. This new format linked progress notes, consultations, and other clinical reports together to create a problem list, each part of which the staff had to address to overcome the illness. The problems ranged from physical issues such as correcting a deformity in a foot to social ones such as finding an alternative living arrangement for a patient no longer able to climb stairs. This approach also provided an audit trail that preserved the logic used by staff in devising solutions to the problems. He also sought to improve the outcomes of care by monitoring and correcting decisions through feedback loops. The heart of the system, named Problem-Oriented Medical Information System (PROMIS), was a series of computerized clinical displays called frames, which clinically aided and taught users as they engaged the system. The data generated by the interaction of users with the system were stored in a computerized patient file. The data were formatted to branch at different decision points, at which users could take the actions proposed in the stored frames or ones of their own choosing. This permitted creative interactions with the information generated not only by physicians but by nurses, pharmacists, and other professional disciplines in the hospital, to all of whom the computer provided the ability to store, retrieve, and analyze data.

Weed anticipated one day linking the system to a national library whose information could be used to update the medical frames and display data. He hoped that the system would fulfill two key goals of patient care: facilitating communication among relevant clinical actors and making it easier for developed clinical standards to be applied by them. Weed wrote:

Patient interviews as we have conducted them, patient records as we have known them, conferences as we have stumbled through them – all must be given a better framework of discipline and form. This can be done through the creative use of modern means of precise and immediate communication. Until we accept the principle that great art does not exist in opposition to structuring and form but requires them, we will never be able to reap the great benefits that the electronic and computer age holds in store. What was precisely communicated on paper by Bach, faithfully performed by Casals, and captured in recordings by modern technology is now available to countless thousands. In the same way, medicine at its best can also be generalized and made available to all if, for each problem, the best current medical standards for defining and treating that problem are available by modern electronic means to each physician. And this aim can and should be achieved in such a way that, as the physician actually records his data and plans the treatments, the very communication tools he uses will have built into them parameters of guidance and the currency of information he needs to define and solve problems. The best talent medicine has must be available to him through computer displays at the time he performs, because it is at the point of integrating knowledge and action that he needs help, not in learning the facts themselves.[28]

Weed applied these tools and ideas of PROMIS clinically at the Medical Center Hospital in Vermont during the 1970s. The results were mixed. One evaluation showed resentment by interns and attending physicians at having to change their style of entering clinical events in the patient record through the computer system. Also concerning them was the intrusion of other staff members, interacting with the system, who seemed to infringe on the physicians' prerogatives. But nurses were enthusiastic, for they enjoyed the greater participation in decision making that their knowledge of and ready access to the system allowed. Pharmacists liked the system for the same reasons. Among physicians, the radiologists, no longer needing to rely on doctors at the bedside to provide reliable clinical data when making imaging requests, particularly appreciated the system.[29]

Another hope in this period was that physicians in their home or office, linked through a computer with patient records and data banks could evaluate evidence and direct therapy at a distance, practicing within a web of telecommunications. Such a vision was a century old. Physicians had reacted this way to the clinical possibilities of the telephone when it was introduced in 1876. With it, they conceived of listening to the heart or lungs of patients at home miles away from them, forestalling the need for a personal visit.[30]

In this modern, automated medical climate of the 1970s and 1980s, it was hoped that the patient record would also enable physicians to more clearly and quickly match the initiation of an action to its outcome, thereby not only providing better care to their patients but also learning from experience. This correlation of action and effect, it will be recalled, had been a goal of reformers of the medical record such as E. A. Codman in the early twentieth century and less well-known doctors, such as one who wrote at this time: "Records are facts that you find, that you filter, that you focus, and then face fearlessly."[31] This also was the viewpoint of Richard Cabot's conferences at MGH, in which clinical actions were evaluated by the yardstick of pathology. Indeed, going even further back to the nineteenth century, this was the rationale of the autopsy itself as advocated by clinicians like Laennec.

When the computer entered the world of medicine in the 1960s, its help in tracking clinical outcomes concerned not only the medical staff. Medicine in this period had become a public institution, bringing a host of new, curious, and powerful eyes to gaze onto the pages of the patient record. At the decade's beginning, decisions at the bedside essentially were private in character. The triad of physician, patient, and family decided the therapy in the confines of professional and legal canons and basically free of the oversight of others. The combination of a successful political effort to broaden the rights of large segments of American society to a federal subsidy for health care (resulting in the 1965 passage of Medicare and Medicaid legislation) and the invention of a new and highly expensive technology of rescue (starting in 1960 with the artificial kidney and creating by mid-decade widespread diffusion of the intensive care unit) by the decade's end had produced a significant consequence: the social oversight of medical care.

Government officials wanted its medical entitlements fairly distributed, provided at high quality, and allocated in a cost-effective manner. Insurance companies, some of which were fiscal intermediates for governmental medical-care programs, became increasingly concerned with the content of practice and the use of resources in caring for patients. In the 1970s and 1980s, payor groups representing business, labor, patients, and consumers expressed growing interest in how medical care was given, which in the 1990s led to the development of managed-care organizations to control medical costs. During this period, professional societies such as the American Medical Association joined with government to oversee the effectiveness of practice, creating, for example, physician standards review organizations. The administrative division of the hospital and other providers like health maintenance organizations (HMOs), with an enlarged responsibility to deal with multiple regulations and payment mechanisms, assumed a correspondingly greater authority. These arrangements gradually led to a dominance of institutional policy making by administrators who, in this respect, overshadowed the professional staff.

Thus, since the time when the Medicare and Medicaid laws were passed, a public medicine has developed whose multiple constituents seek to assess the way in which technology is used, mainly from the perspectives of cost and quality. This assessment is possible only by knowing what is done clinically, which makes creating a patient record a pivotal element in setting policy and governing practice.

But as records became vehicles that institutions sought to use in monitoring and managing staff actions for quality, quantity, and costs of care, they were found wanting: the human skills and technology available were not quite ready for the task. In 1989 Jerome Grossman, president of the New England Medical Center, reflected on his experience with this issue at the beginning of the 1970s:

[during my] first foray into using data to influence physician practice patterns in the start-up phase of a staff model HMO, [I] developed an automated medical record system for the HMO, believing that physicians would use clinical information in aggregate form to develop cost-effective protocols for treating patients. (Their motive: they were participating in a pre-paid medical plan where the goals had shifted from more units/patients to a goal of judicious use of services to each patient.) But the information in the medical record was only a limited part of the data needed to make cost decisions about patient care. A medical record system does not include the financial information that is critical to this decision-making process. Also, the physicians had no way to assess each individual service's contribution to the outcomes.[32]

Grossman reported that things had improved by 1989. By that time, he had helped develop an information system "integrating clinical and financial information, and creating a management control system for planning, budgeting, and periodic monitoring" of health services and administrative transactions, which became the principal means of budgeting and monitoring care in the hospital. Here, and in other clinical settings, the record showed when practice patterns fell within guidelines established by the institution for resource use, by federal regulations, by insurance companies' payment standards, and by the multiple other public and private parties concerned with the particular clinical actions as well as the basic goals of medicine.

Many of the developments were considered in a 1991 report by the National Academy of Science's Institute of Medicine on the possibilities of a computer-based patient record. The report argued that to automate the form and content of the paper record without redefining the goals of its use would merely lock its deficiencies into any new system created. The goals set by the report for a computerized patient record, a number of which had been articulated in the 1970s by Lawrence Weed, were providing clinicians with accurate data on the evolving state of the patient, giving practitioners reminders and alerts about interventions needed by the patient, providing clinical decision support to clinicians and linking them to reservoirs of medical knowledge in its vast literature, storing patient data (its classic use) in formats that better organized and displayed it such as with video and picture graphics, offering an electronic mail capability to transfer data between practitioners, and giving nonclinical users such as payors and government agencies information they needed to carry out their health care functions.[33]

Progress toward the goals stated in the 1991 document was slow. Another Institute of Medicine report published in 2000 on ways to reduce medical errors and the resultant injuries and deaths they caused in the health system was still calling for action to develop standard ways of recording medical data in patient records and improving means of linking and using information systems to provide better and safer care. A computerized record was essential to meeting these goals. It could diminish clinical errors, for example, by providing access to needed data without delay and dependable assurance that ordered therapies were given. But the report declared: "Despite the computer-based patient record being 'almost here' for 45 years, it has still not arrived."[34]

That judgment remained valid as the new century progressed. Legislation to make government support available to facilitate the use of electronic health information by medical institutions and providers remained stalled in Congress, despite intense lobbying from President George W. Bush in his 2004 State of the Union address, when he called for a "health information technology infrastructure [that] reduces health-care costs resulting from inefficiency, medical errors, inappropriate care and incomplete information." This recommendation included adopting the electronic health record (EHR), which a government report issued in 2005 asserted could reduce the cost of health care by as much as 20 percent a year. "Or can it?" wrote Jason Sidorow in *Health Affairs* a year later: "A considerable body of evidence suggests that widespread adoption of the EHR increases health care costs." Cost was a major factor influencing the adoption of the EHR by doctors, which, like congressional action on it, has been slow. A national survey of physicians providing ambulatory care in office settings, published in 2008, found only four percent had an electronic record system with features that made it "fully functional," that is, storing and retrieving data gained from and about patients, facilitating medical orders, and supplying information to guide decision making. Thirteen percent of doctors had a less complete system that nonetheless gave them basic practice support. Inhibiting adoption were its capital costs, and allied concerns about investment return, capability to serve practice needs, and vulnerability to obsolescence. A parallel survey of American hospitals published a year later displayed similar results. Fewer than two percent had electronic record systems defined by study authors as "comprehensive," using criteria analogous to those applied to the systems found in doctors' offices. Fewer than eight percent had systems that performed a core of these functions. But many hospitals selectively chose particular tasks, such as medication ordering, to be formatted electronically. Like physicians, hospitals cited purchase and maintenance costs as the predominant barriers to adopting the electronic record and financial gain as a major incentive to have it. However, the reservations about the technology introduced by monetary issues were compounded by disagreement among users about its performance. While some reported that electronic health records diminished errors, increased productivity, and facilitated cost-effective practice, others dissented from these claims.[35]

But as policy makers and health care experts debated the advantages and problems of computerized records, an unrelated external event influenced the outcome. To meliorate the ravages of a major and deepening recession, in early 2009 President Barack Obama and Congress produced economic stimulus legislation, the American Recovery and Reinvestment Act. It was designed not only to create jobs and meet immediate public needs, but also to advance fields of development important to the national interest. And one of the chosen areas to promote and subsidize was an electronically-linked health system. For this purpose the act created an administrative apparatus to advance and oversee such a system, and incentives to induce doctors and hospitals to join the effort: notably, nineteen billion dollars of assistance to help them computerize health records, but payment penalties for patient care given through the government-run Medicare and Medicaid programs by providers who continued to use paper records several years after the assistance program began. While the federal subsidy is a small portion of the funds needed to establish a nation-wide electronic record system, the act tangibly solidified and proclaimed a public interest in having the technology used, and thus increased the prospect of placing it into the daily routines of American health care. However, beyond the matter of financing its cost, it is crucial to ensure that the system's health providers receive one of the technology's greatest benefits – a rapid and comprehensive gathering of health information from the multiple sources of care given to patients made accessible wherever they are. National standards and policies that spur development and purchase of electronic record systems capable of being linked, therefore, are essential. Without this ability, as a U.S. secretary of health and human services put it: "Systems will be isolated; data undecipherable; health quality unimproved. If we're going to build a 21st-century health infrastructure, we need to do it strategically, continuing the careful work on harmonized standards that will create one nationwide, interoperable system. That's the only way to make an investment in health IT produce value for providers and patients and improve the quality of care overall."[36] Significantly, the recovery act advanced this goal by requiring the development of such standards and implementation criteria.

These events heighten the attention that should be given to the influence of the electronic record on clinical fact-finding, reporting, and analysis, areas in which some doctors report improvement and others troubling behavior. As they used and received electronic records, for example, two Harvard clinicians discerned physicians and residents who cut and pasted portions of notes made by other doctors about a patient's medical history into their own examination note, which the authors labeled "a form of clinical plagiarism." Further, they found doctors who integrated information from past evaluations that they themselves had made of patients into current notes about them. While the pressure of burdensome clinical demands, the appropriateness of repeating certain aspects of medical evaluations, and the need to satisfy billing requirements partly explained such behavior, the clinicians were particularly troubled by the reflection of a conceptual hazard that electronic formatting and processing of clinical data created for medicine. As they state: "Writing in a personal and independent way forces us to think and formulate our ideas. Notes that are meant to be focused have become voluminous and templated, distracting from the key cognitive work of providing care. Such charts may satisfy the demands of third-party payors, but they are the product of a word-processor, not of physicians' thoughtful review and analysis. They may be 'efficient' for the purpose of documentation but not creative thinking." These authors pointed also to the penchant of electronic systems to gather and drop into the record hoards of data without selectivity, which made finding relevant facts more difficult, and described doctors who used scarce time with patients fixed on their computer screen, typing in data, or whose inquiries were excessively dictated and limited by filling in the standardized information template of the electronic record.[37]

Such problems reflect the ability of a powerful technology to channel users along particular paths of inquiry and action, which may not always achieve clinical outcomes that best serve patients' interest.

In the midst of discussions on automating patient records, a growing effort to encourage consumers to create their own health history received a boost in 2007 and 2008 when the major information-technology firms Microsoft and Google announced separate plans to offer consumers online repositories in which to store their health information and create personal health records.[38] These and other companies urged consumers to place health data into electronic storage bins (which they provided) and ask multiple practitioners who treated them at different times and in different places to assist filling in their medical history and making it up to date. This would give consumers an alternative to health providers as the keepers of their medical information, as well as continuous access to their record as they moved from place to place. As one doctor noted:

If personally controlled records take off – and despite the enthusiasm of proponents, there is no assurance that they will – the electronic records maintained by physicians and hospitals will be only one component of a larger Web-based information system with national interoperability standards, in which patients increasingly control their own health data. Patients will be able to download their data from medical records, laboratories, pharmacies, and insurance-claims databases, and add data, such as measurements of weight or blood pressure. Without carrying paper records, they will be able to share data with multiple doctors, an emergency department, or family members as necessary; renew prescriptions; manage their fitness, diet, or a chronic disease such as diabetes or congestive heart failure; communicate with people with similar health problems; or find clinical trials to participate in.[39]

The concept of having a personal health record is another indicator of the reach of consumers for authority over their treatment by the health system. But the downside of depending on corporations to secure intensely private data is a feature of the movement to the EHR that must be addressed. With so many people now having access to a highly personal aspect of an individual's life – the story of illness and recovery as recounted in patient records – can this information remain confidential? Respect for confidentiality was first cogently expressed in the

Hippocratic oath, which, to be emphatic, called communications from patients "holy secrets."[40] For the promise of confidentiality encouraged patients to be truthful to and trusting of doctors, thus improving the likelihood of successful care and medical relationships. This explains the concern of doctors about preserving the confidentiality of exchanges with patients if accounts of them were placed in hospital records, which had held back the reform of record keeping in the early twentieth century. Accordingly, doctors kept these records safely, if incompletely, in office files and memory. But as the century progressed and written documentation and hospital residence of records became necessary and accepted, their openness to the gaze of increasing numbers of social and administrative personnel and specialized medical staff doing care and research grew. This stirred public concern over their confidentiality and, as a consequence, resulted in federal legislation.

In 2003 the Health Insurance Portability and Accountability Act (HIPAA), legislation passed by the U.S. Congress several years earlier, became operative. It created national standards that improved the access of patients to see and request corrections of mistakes in their medical records; it placed clear limits on the way health plans and doctors could use or share patient information for purposes unrelated to direct patient care such as research, insurance reimbursement, and marketing; and it required institutions with access to health data such as hospitals and medical schools to train personnel in privacy procedures and issues. But despite the law's good intentions, implementing HIPAA rules generated burdensome paperwork and bureaucratic procedures. This often directed the focus of health providers and organizations more to documenting the fact that rules were being followed than to inculcating in them the social and ethical significance of confidential medical transactions. In addition, the rules did not prevent security lapses at insurance companies, hospitals, and agencies of government from compromising the privacy of health data on hundreds of thousands of people – an issue that has further slowed the adoption of EHRs. The problem is driven by the data's growing commercial value. As the coordinator of the group Coalition for Patient Privacy observed: "Health IT without privacy is an excellent way for companies to establish a gold mine of information that can be used to increase profits, promote expensive drugs, cherry-pick patients who are cheaper to insure and market directly to consumers."[41] Of course, material in the paper record is at risk of being accessed and used by those who should not, and in ways that are wrong. But the information it holds can be broadcast neither as widely nor as rapidly as that stored in its electronic successor, or as readily abstracted for use.

The issues of disclosure and confidentiality of data in the medical record have not only ethical but legal dimensions as well. In the 1970s, as ethical controversy concerning matters of practice such as the use of life-sustaining technology grew, the courts increasingly entered clinical domains to resolve disputes, notably marked by the Karen Ann Quinlan case (see Chapter 4). In such disputes, and in the burgeoning number of malpractice claims, the patient record provided judges and juries with a view of what was thought and of what was done. This led some physicians to compose records as much to provide an acceptable account to forestall legal problems as to document facts to resolve medical problems, an aspect of behavior that has come to be known as defensive medicine. There is a benefit to this action: a more detailed and carefully written record. But this has a significant negative influence on the record: diminished authenticity. A motive to write the story of the patient's illness and therapy with an eye to self-protection introduces inescapable distortions into clinical reasoning and weakens the record's credibility. The chief of a hospital service in 1990 noted that, in contemporary medicine, there sometimes was "more worrying about what to document than its therapeutic goal."[42]

A further challenge for the patient record is the adequacy of its text to fulfill its multiple uses. For the record must at once serve regulatory, fiscal, scientific, and clinical purposes, as well as the personal needs of the patient. Historically, the record mainly has addressed the needs of medical staff. It has focused on the technical facts of the illness and at its best portrayed the hypotheses and logic underlying clinical actions. But it is unlikely that a discussion formulated to meet clinical objectives can also fulfill the information needs of the public, particularly as it seeks inputs from doctors in creating personal health records. On this issue, the experience in producing consent forms for research subjects provides guidance. It demonstrates the difficulties of converting technical discourse to vernacular language and the dangers of confusion or false impression when failing to do so. We are thus left with significant questions: Can a single account of illness serve multiple regulatory, fiscal, medical, and patient needs and deal with the privacy issue? Not well. Are different versions of the health record needed for its several constituents? Probably so. Will computerizing records produce the capability for and generate an interest in this needed reformatting? Technically, yes, but a major obstacle is the human work and thought needed to reformat medical data to serve multiple uses.

In the United States, the patient record began as an instrument to portray the experiences and results of treatment to practitioners of medicine for the purposes of patient care. In the nineteenth century, as medicine became more complex, the documenting of medical actions served wider purposes, such as providing statistics that proved to the donors and overseers of hospitals the quality of care given within them.

In the early twentieth century, the record began to assume the role of integrator. As specialization directed the view of physicians and other medical staff to increasingly circumscribed perspectives on illness, the record was the only technology that revealed their collective actions as they gathered together to practice under the roofs of modern hospitals. At this time, the record started to shed its personal but not its private character. Thus, by the 1920s, professional accrediting agencies like ACS singled it out as a key indicator of whether standards of practice were being met by physicians and hospitals. But this examination was carried out by fellow professionals and not social others.

In the 1960s, as American medicine changed its fundamental character from a private to a public enterprise, the record of its activities became essential to social institutions that assumed basic roles in its governance. And these events have turned the record into a contradictory hybrid: a confidential and public document. The integrative burdens the record bears have become ever greater as the constituencies it knits together grow more diverse. For the record serves not only the clinical world but also the managers of health organizations who need it to control costs, evaluate regulatory compliance, assess quality, prevent legal penalty, and facilitate ethical decisions, as well as the consumer owners of its content as they gain increasing authority and responsibility as stewards of their health.[43] Thus, the record is the principal means to understand and monitor how the entire enterprise of medicine functions.

Despite this crucial unifying role, caution is needed in the face of excessive expectations about how transformative the EHR can be. It improves many aspects of health care but diminishes some, too. And while its wider use will improve the effectiveness and efficiency of the practice, organization, and governance of medicine, the EHR cannot, as many believe, fundamentally reshape its care or cost. For this, more is needed, a matter that is considered subsequently.

6

PUTTING TECHNOLOGIES
ON TRIAL

From Bloodletting to Antibiotics to
the Oregon Initiative

Each day, the media bombard the public with claims about scientific advances capable of soothing ills from headaches to stomach pain; enhancing the ability to exercise, think, and work; and preventing problems from aging to weight gain. Health providers receive a similarly relentless cluster of messages in their journals, clothed in the garb of scientific statements backed by mountains of numbers and tables to substantiate an idea, at least until disputed, disproved, and replaced by another. Only sleep relieves the burden of knowing what or whom to believe, until an alarm clock propels us back into the stream of claims and promises the new day will bring. The scientific community that generates the innovations around us has struggled with the issue of how to evaluate its work. And one of the earliest and most significant efforts to do this was applied to assess the longest continually used therapy in Western medicine – bloodletting.

A lancet to pierce veins and a bowl to catch blood constitute the essential technologies of bloodletting. There are records of its use at least 2,500 years ago by Hippocrates, and it was a therapeutic mainstay of Galen, the Greek physician who wrote comprehensively on the theoretical basis and practical applications of bloodletting in the second century of the modern era.[1] Galen's ideas on this subject, as on other medical issues, influenced the practice of doctors for more than 1,500 years. Galen asserted that the main reason for bloodletting was to rid the body of excess matter. Such matter was generated when reactions to the social and physical environments of living, for example, diet and climate, led to an increase in one of the four humors, the basic building blocks of the body, and produced symptoms of illness. Elimination of the excess matter restored humoral equilibrium and health.

Until the nineteenth century, imbalance of the humors and the restoration of their normal proportions in the body was the main theoretical explanation for how illness was caused and health was regained. Since bloodletting was a central means of reestablishing the natural balance of the humors, its long-term dominance as a therapy was ensured.

Although the basic technique of bloodletting is simple – open a vein, let out some blood, and stanch the wound – its overall complexity is great. First, the patient was evaluated as an individual, a difficult undertaking because people differ greatly in their temperaments, past and present ways of living, physical makeup, and so forth. The variations, it was believed, influenced the balance of the humors in their body. Then, for given symptoms, one had to judge the total amount of blood to be removed, from which site or sites in the body should it be taken, how much blood to let from each place, how often the bleeding should be done, how to adjust the volume bled and site selection as the symptoms changed, and so forth. It could take years to knowledgeably link the theoretical considerations of when to use bloodletting to the symptomatic considerations dictating its application to individual patients.

In some periods, bloodletting was carried to an extreme, such as from the late eighteenth to the early nineteenth century, when Benjamin Rush, one of America's most famous colonial doctors and the only physician to sign the Declaration of Independence, was an ardent advocate of the therapy. Rush developed a theory that all illnesses were manifestations of one basic condition – excessive excitation of arterial walls. He declared that the greatest arterial irritant was blood, and therefore, more than any other therapy, its removal relaxed the arteries and helped defeat illness. He praised bloodletting's rapid effects, ease of use, and safety. He thought as much as 80 percent of a person's blood could be removed without harm and argued against withholding bleeding in conditions thought by his medical colleagues to warrant restraint, such as patients in whom it caused fainting, whose condition worsened after several bleedings, or who persistently used it when well in the hope of preventing disease. While Rush and some others applied bloodletting to excess, it remained a mainstay of therapy and was the most common surgical procedure performed in America during Revolutionary times (Figure 13).[2]

By the mid-1830s James Jackson, a respected physician at Massachusetts General Hospital, could declare that "if anything may be

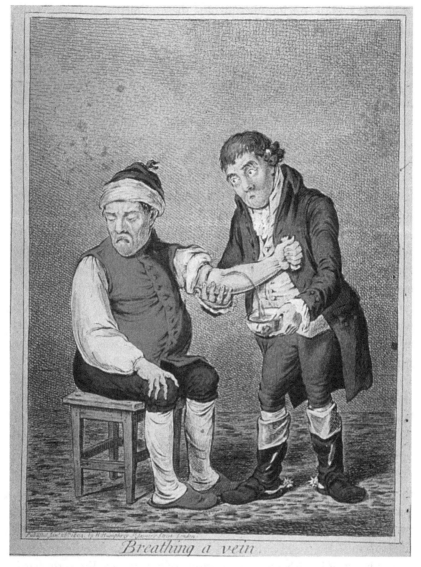

Figure 13. "Breathing a Vein," by James Gillray, depicting bloodletting therapy. London, H. Humphrey, 1804. Courtesy of the National Library of Medicine.

regarded as settled in the treatment of diseases," it was the usefulness of bloodletting in the large and important class of illness then called inflammations, particularly as they afflicted the organs of the chest.[3] He focused his comments on this class and place of illness in the preface to an 1835 book on bloodletting for these ailments, written by the innovative French doctor Pierre Louis.

Louis had decided on a career as a private practitioner at age thirty-two and as a prelude to this choice reviewed the scientific basis of the medicine of his time. Disappointed in what he found, Louis changed direction and became a medical scientist, determined to take the description of illness in patients to a new level of exactness. He painstakingly extracted from patients accounts of their life that described how they felt when well and the character and sequence of symptoms they experienced when overtaken by illness. He used a similar level of precision in his physical examinations and, if the patients died, in their autopsies. When he had accumulated an adequate group of cases, Louis used the evidence to make generalizations about the development of illness. With medical colleagues in Paris, he formed the Society of Medical Observation to discuss and compare experiences and ideas. The objectivity with which Louis studied the natural history of diseases and devised concepts upon which to base their diagnoses and prognoses was applied to the study of therapy and exhibited in his work on bloodletting.

Louis starts his book by revealing the anxiety of the innovator who challenges established doctrine, which in this case is no less than the basic therapy of medicine. "The results of my researches on the effects of bloodletting in inflammation are so little in accordance with the general opinion, that it is not without a degree of hesitation I have decided to publish them." He describes analyzing his initial data and how, thinking they must be wrong, decided to start over. Again he got the same results, and convinced that "he could no longer doubt their correctness," he determined to "state them to the reader as they at first presented themselves to me."[4]

The heart of Louis's work is a critique of experience. From the earliest medical writings to Louis's own time, experience had been the basis of determining the credibility of evidence and the wisdom of action. Louis defines the two fundamental sources of experience. One was the medical texts of revered predecessors or famous contemporaries whose pronouncements doctors accepted as facts. A second was the conclusions physicians drew from remembered outcomes of their own encounters with patients or the witnessed interventions of others.

Louis uses cases taken from texts on bloodletting to show the limitations of expert-based experience. One text, for example, raises the questions of whether a patient having the lung disorder pleurisy should be bled from the arm or foot and if the bleeding performed should be from the side of the body in which the disorder resided. The author's response is given: "Opinions have been hitherto divided on this point; but the voice of experience seems at last to have declared... from the arm of the painful side. The practice of Triller may serve as a guide in this particular.... He comments upon a violent pleurisy of the right side, which had existed with severity for three days; blood was abstracted from the left arm which was not indicated. Triller bled the patient from the right arm and all went well." To Louis, this response displays little more than authority worship: "The author's mind is so preoccupied with Triller's doctrines, that he does not perceive that two bleedings may be more efficacious than a single one; and he draws a conclusion in favor of Triller's doctrine."[5]

Louis also questions the value of direct physician experience to justify interventions, unaccompanied by a methodical analysis of actions and outcomes. He notes: "When physicians are called to attend on a patient, if after having agreed upon the character and kind of disease, one of them differs from his colleagues in regard to the treatment proposed, what does he do to sustain his views?... He urges the preference of his own plan, on the ground that he has seen it more often successful than any other proposed."[6] Louis endeavors to redefine the meaning and the usefulness of experience in medicine by wedding it to the collection and analysis of facts at the bedside, categorized according to their similarity and critically compared. His great achievement would be to develop and prove the validity of a new mode of making comparisons from which the data to ground practice is gained.

Louis approached his task by collecting cases in three diseases (affecting the lungs, face, and tonsils) that he frequently encountered in his hospital work and whose primary treatment was bloodletting. He chose the cases from patients of his in perfect health before their first symptoms appeared and who thus entered the realm of disease from the same starting place. At the center of his work was the creation of tables, which group and display the comparative experiences and outcomes of the patients he treated. For example, in one table, he compares patients according to when in the course of their illness they were first bled, how often treatment was repeated, and how long their illness lasted. In another table, he compares time of bleeding with the patients' age. He also evaluates in a similar manner the influence of bloodletting on major aspects of the studied disorders such as pain, pulse rate, temperature, and so forth.

He concludes from his work that bloodletting had little influence on the progress of the three diseases he evaluated. It mattered not if patients were bled copiously and often, or bled once and sparely. He attributed the cases in which improvement occurred during the hospital stay either to an erroneous diagnosis or to the fact that the bloodletting was done on patients who sought treatment late in the course of the disease, which had almost reached its end. While the influence of bloodletting was proved generally wanting by this research, Louis believed it had a few good effects and a limited place in treating the diseases investigated.

The basis of Louis's studies is a method of analysis that requires an investigator to collect a sufficient number of cases to compare the influence of treatment on patients. The key objection raised by his critics was the impossibility of gathering a group of patients sufficiently similar to make such comparisons. Louis acknowledged the problem but proposed a way out. Since the formation of a group of identical patients was impossible, the creation of a large-enough pool of similar patients caused their differences to mutually cancel one another. His method did not erase differences; it supposed them. Louis concludes: "Between him who counts his facts, grouped according to their resemblance, in order to learn what value he can attach to therapeutic agents, and him who does not count, but who contents himself with repeating *more or less, rarely or frequently*; there is the difference of truth and error; of a thing clear and truly scientific on one hand, and of something vague and worthless on the other: for what place can be assigned in science to that which is uncertain? ... *If then there is a means of embodying the experience of ages, it is the numerical method.*"[7] Although, as shall be shown, other clinicians before Louis introduced a comparative perspective and numerical dimension into the evaluation of treatments, making such analyses the fundamental means of testing therapy and elevating the significance of numerical analysis in determining scientific facts was Louis's essential accomplishment.

As noted, Louis discerned that the key to assembling a group of patients on whom to test therapy was to create a cluster large enough to have their differences cancel out. But he did not have the mathematical capability needed to formally explore the question of just how many individuals constituted a group large enough to statistically prove a point (a lacuna that a colleague, Jules Gavarret, helped fill in an 1840 book on medical statistics).[8] Nor did Louis fully recognize two potential sources of bias in his work: the influence of his own hand in selecting the patients studied and in observing the effects of treatment on them, each of which could have been affected by his hopes for a particular outcome.

A time-honored approach to overcoming bias in situations involving selection is the drawing or casting of lots, in the form of objects such as sticks, pebbles, or dice. The basis of confidence in them resides in their ability to resolve issues through chance and thus a random mechanism, which equalizes the prospects for a particular outcome among alternative choices or claimants and removes responsibility for it from the involved parties. The lot has been used since biblical times to divide land, allocate tasks, decide rewards, choose rulers, pick jurors, draft soldiers, make personal decisions, and settle disputes.[9]

In premodern medicine, lots were used on occasion to ensure that the division of patients in tests of different treatments resulted in the formation of like groups. For example, in 1662 the Flemish doctor Jean Baptiste van Helmont proposed an experiment to determine whether his therapy, or bloodletting and purging, was the best treatment for fevers:

"If ye speak truth, Oh ye Schools, that ye can cure any kind of Fevers without evacuation, but will not fear of a worse relapse; come down to the contest ye Humorists: Let us take out of the Hospitals, out of the Camps, or from elsewhere, 200, or 500 poor People, that have Fevers, Pleurisies, etc. Let us divide them in Halfes, let us cast lots, that one half of them may fall to my share and the other to yours; I will cure them without bloodletting and sensible evacuation; but do you do as ye know ... we shall see how many Funerals both of us shall have: But let the reward of the contention or wager, be 300 Florens, deposited on both sides: here your business is decided."[10]

While it is not known whether van Helmont's challenge was accepted, he embraced the use of chance allocation to create similar groups of patients upon whom to compare therapies.

A second early example of an effort to create like comparison groups in medical research occurred in 1747, when James Lind developed a strategy to test different treatments for scurvy. As a ship's surgeon, Lind witnessed the terrible conditions under which sailors lived during voyages that often took months or years. He claimed that the world's navies lost "more of their men by sickness than the sword," as a result of unsanitary living quarters and inadequate diet. The worst illness afflicting crew was scurvy, which caused pain, exhaustion, internal bleeding, and death. In one example of its devastation, an expedition to sail round the world that left England in 1740 with a crew of about 2,000 men returned four years later with 638. Most died from scurvy.

Lind had an idea that scurvy might be prevented by a dietary intervention and tested it on a voyage in 1747. His research subjects were twelve sailors who displayed similar symptoms of scurvy, occupied the same living space on the ship, and received the same daily diet. He thus endeavored to bring together similarly affected patients living in similar circumstances as the prelude to dividing them among the treatments. Lind was aware of the generic problem of selection bias and dealt with it by striving to create a group of like subjects among whom to allocate the remedies he wished to study. Accordingly, he separated the twelve sailors into six pairs and assigned a different daily treatment to each. The therapies compared were a quart of cider; sweet oil of vitriol (now called ether); vinegar; seawater; a paste of garlic, radish, Peru balsam, and myrrh; and oranges and lemons. By the end of six days the pair who had consumed the citrus fruits remained healthy while the others became ill.[11,12]

Lind did not view the cause of scurvy and its prevention by eating lemons and oranges in nutritional terms. He thought its source was blocked perspiration ducts caused by the damp air of ships and that the citruses broke up toxic materials that prevented perspiration from leaving the body. However, the success of his therapy was dramatic and later championed by the explorer James Cook. In 1795 the British Navy ordered its fleet to provide a daily ration of lemon juice to sailors, and within two years scurvy had virtually disappeared as a shipboard problem. However, it took another seventy years for private shipping companies to fully adopt Lind's findings.[13]

While one technique to create like comparison groups was the use of random assignment methods such as lots, a second used a bias-free and consistent means to assemble the groups such as strict alternation. An example of this occurred in a mid-nineteenth-century trial of a remedy to prevent scarlet fever among orphans housed at the Royal Military Asylum in Chelsea, England. The investigator was the surgeon Thomas Balfour, who in this study also showed the value of comparison groups in establishing the true action of medical remedies:

"There were 151 boys of whom I had tolerably satisfactory evidence that they had not had scarlatina; I divided them in two sections, taking them alternately from the list, to prevent the imputation of selection. To the first section (76) I gave belladonna: to the second (75) I gave none; the result was that two in each section were attacked by the disease. The numbers are too small to justify deductions as to the prophylactic power of belladonna, but the observation is good, because it shows how apt we are to be misled by imperfect observation. Had I given the remedy to all the boys, I should probably have attributed to it the cessation of the epidemic."[14]

After the 1920s, studies in the medical literature increasingly apply means such as lotteries or alternation to create a dependable experimental structure through which to evaluate therapies.[15]

Concurrent with the evolution of techniques to control the bias of selection in putting together experimental groups of patients were efforts to control the bias of the investigators who create and observe experiments and the patients and practitioners who participate in them and report the effects of therapies. This bias is largely the result of the investigator's and subject's expectations about the treatments being evaluated and foreknowledge of their identity. Possibly the first and a dramatic example of efforts to overcome such observer bias was the evaluation of the therapeutic effectiveness of mesmerism by a French royal commission led by the American representative to France, Benjamin Franklin.

Franz Anton Mesmer, who lived from 1735 to 1815, believed he had the ability to harness a natural force that he called animal magnetism, a power that a mesmerist could either transmit himself or invest in material objects such as mirrors and thus make the remedy accessible to patients at any time (Figure 14). Mesmer's success, particularly among the French elite, produced consternation in established medical circles,

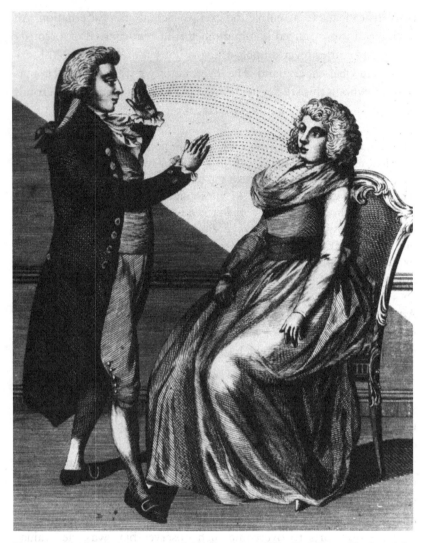

Figure 14. A patient being mesmerized. Reprinted from Sibley E. A Key to Physic and the Occult Sciences. London, 1794. Courtesy of the National Library of Medicine.

which in 1784 led Louis XVI to appoint the commission of inquiry to study its value. The commission was to determine whether Mesmer's results were produced by the mental influence of the patient's belief in the therapy or by physical powers unaffected by the perceptions of patients. The commissioners developed a series of trials on single individuals, which removed practitioner influence or patient awareness from the outcome of treatment by the use of masking methods. They found in all of their tests that masking eliminated the influence of mesmerism and that sham treatments had the same effect as real ones. For example, in one experiment, a cooperating mesmerist was separated from female patients in an adjoining room by a paper curtain over a doorway. When told (falsely) that they were receiving mesmeric therapy, the women reported feeling its typical sensations. But when they were not informed of being mesmerized (they were waiting for the treatment), they felt nothing. From this and other experiments, the commission determined that animal magnetism was not real and that the effects of Mesmer's treatment were creations of his patients' belief in it.[16]

An effort to deal with both selection and observer bias is found in an experiment conducted from 1911 to 1914 by the German scientist Adolf Bingle on a newly developed antitoxin treatment for diphtheria. The initial hope for the success of the antitoxin had given way to disappointment, as the problems of administering it at the right time in the disease and the different virulence of diphtheria from season to season made evaluation of its effectiveness difficult and raised skepticism about its value. "To make as objective a test as possible," Bingle wrote, he assigned 937 patients in an alternating fashion to the diphtheria antitoxin serum or to an inactive horse serum as a decoy or placebo, with neither the attending physicians nor the patients aware of which substance was given. Bingle thus combined a means of eliminating selection bias and observer bias in both patients and participating practitioners (with the exception of Bingle) in the experiment. He called his procedure a blind method.[17] This experiment demonstrated the value of a technique that created dependably comparable study groups joined to an assessment process that promoted an objective reporting of study results.

At this time, a person appeared on the scene who became a transformative figure in clinical research, Austin Bradford Hill. Hill contracted tuberculosis during service in the First World War and used his convalescence to study economics. He then took a position that brought him into contact with Major Greenwood, a leading British statistician who in 1927 became the first professor of epidemiology and public health at the London School of Hygiene and was a prominent figure in the government-sponsored Medical Research Council. Greenwood was connected to the Hill family, having been a student of Hill's father during earlier work in physiology. The younger Hill studied statistical methods with Greenwood and others and became a member of the London School faculty in 1933. Two years later, a book on research design and statistics appeared, *The Design of Experiments*, by R. A. Fisher, a British statistician and an acquaintance of Hill. It portrayed randomization as a crucial means of dealing with the uncertainty and variability inherent in biological phenomena. The ideas presented in the work stemmed from experiments undertaken in agriculture that involved comparison of grain yields by seeding experimental plots through a random method. Fisher maintained that such random assignment removed the biases of investigators and created objective results. While not directly involving work on human subjects, the book contributed additional standing in the period to the scientific significance of randomization as a research technique, and to medical statisticians themselves as important collaborators in research studies.[18,19]

In 1937 one of Britain's leading medical journals, the *Lancet* asked Hill to write articles for it on the use of statistics in medicine, which he did and soon turned into the book *Principles of Medical Statistics*. Hill maintained in these writings that a crucial problem in the experimenter's work alleviated by statistical methods was to ensure "that we are really comparing like with like, and that we have not overlooked a relevant factor which is present in Group A and absent in Group B."[20] Hill's work was aimed at a dilemma encountered by physicians of this time trying to understand the effects of their remedies on patients but stymied by an age-old problem. If patients didn't recover or died, obviously the applied remedy had failed. But if they got better, how to determine whether they were healed by the remedy or by nature? To overcome this difficulty, investigators compared patients given a new therapy with a similar group of patients whom they had treated with different measures in the past, a so-called historical control group. But such a comparison, doctors of this period complained, stumbled against the problem of group dissimilarity: how to prove that past and present patient groups were enough alike in the way the illness was biologically expressed in them and in the economic and social circumstances that influenced their reactions to treatment.[21] Hill argued for the groups studied in an experiment to be formed of patients in the present and chosen through a chance-based process.

From the writing of his book and the articles on statistics until the end of the Second World War, the idea of conducting clinical trials based on comparing like groups formed and evaluated through procedures that eliminated basic biases filled Hill's thoughts.[22] He had several opportunities to carry out such research but only in nonclinical settings. For instance, in this period, he helped design a Medical Research Council study to evaluate a vaccine for whooping cough, which used random means to allocate it. Also at this time, several other investigators were adopting bias-free measures in designing experiments. The Medical Research Council itself conducted a study in 1944 that used alternation as a means of forming groups to test the antibiotic patulin to treat the common cold. In that same year, an investigation of tuberculosis therapies at the Mayo Clinic in Minnesota involved both a chance-based process to allocate patients and had physicians who read their X-rays masked concerning what therapy patients in the experiment received.[23] In 1945 Hill succeeded his teacher Greenwood as professor of medical statistics at the University of London and as director of what would become the Statistical Research Unit of the Medical Research Council.[24] His role there put him into a more favorable position to influence the clinical test he had hoped for. The opportunity would soon come from America.

The antibiotic streptomycin had been discovered two years earlier by the student Albert Schatz in the laboratory of the eminent scientist Selman Waksman at Rutgers University in New Jersey. It had proved highly effective against tuberculosis infections in laboratory animals and later in preliminary human trials at the Mayo Clinic. In 1946 the British government asked the council to conduct clinical trial of streptomycin. By this time production of the drug in the United States created a supply large enough for patients to get it without enrolling in a research program. While there was much more to learn about the drug, this situation made further clinical trials of it in the United States difficult.[25]

But the situation in the United Kingdom was different. The war had exhausted the dollar supply of the British Treasury, and it could afford to purchase only a small quantity of streptomycin. This made it possible for Hill to argue "that in this situation it would not be immoral to make a trial – it would be immoral *not* to make a trial since the opportunity would never rise again (streptomycin would be synthesized [in the United Kingdom], there would soon be plenty of it, and so on)." At a November 1946 meeting of the council's Streptomycin Clinical Trials Committee and in other forums, the committee's secretary, the physician Philip D'Arcy Hart, supported Hill on the need to make "a really good controlled trial" to determine an effective treatment for tuberculosis. "He argued from the medical point of view," Hill writes, "while I was arguing from the statistical."[26]

After allocating much of its store of streptomycin to treat two rapidly fatal forms of tuberculosis (the miliary and meningeal types), the council released the remainder to treat a type of tuberculosis (acute progressive bilateral pulmonary tuberculosis) in which the standard therapy involving collapse of the lungs was unsuited and bed rest was left as the only alternative. To eliminate as many variations as possible, the trials committee limited the subjects chosen to those whose disease was recently acquired and bacteriologically proven. Since the total number of patients recruited for the trial needed to be small, it initially set the age of subjects at fifteen to twenty-five years. Ultimately, 107 patients entered the trial.

Determination of whether a patient would be given streptomycin and bed rest or bed rest alone was accomplished by a series of random numbers Hill drew up, and from which were created sealed envelopes into which a card bearing an *S* (for the streptomycin and bed rest arm) or *C* (for the bed rest alone control arm) was inserted. After acceptance of a patient by the selection committee and before admission to one of three hospitals collaborating in the study, an appropriately numbered envelope was opened at the central office of the trial, revealing to which arm of the study the patient would go. The data were then given to the medical office of the admitting hospital. Thus, study coordinators, clinicians, and patients could not influence the selection process. Previous efforts to create comparable groups on whom to test therapies had failed to recognize that the knowledge of the group to which a patient would go could influence the selection of patients, for example, by clinicians worried about the welfare of a particular patient.[27] As Chalmers writes: "Bradford Hill's explicit recognition of allocation concealment represents the most recent substantive milestone in the history of efforts to create unbiassed groups in therapeutic experiments which goes back over three centuries."[28]

An ethical issue that the Streptomycin Clinical Trials Committee had to face in the study design concerned the form of the streptomycin therapy: it was to be given through four daily injections into the muscles over a four-month period. How, then, to create a parallel treatment for the control group? The investigators rejected as excessively harmful the idea of giving the controls similar intramuscular injections of saline for so long a time. This meant the study would lose the appearance of equality of treatment to its subjects and investigators, and increase the introduction of bias in interpreting its results. However, the radiologists who read the chest X-rays of patients in both groups to determine treatment effects would have no knowledge of the groups to which patients belonged, and the committee believed that this meliorated the absence of parallel-looking placebo treatment. Looking back on this study, the contemporary designer of experiments Richard Doll agrees: "The response to treatment could be assessed objectively without it: psychological factors would have had little impact on such a serious disease."[29] Hill reflected on this dilemma also, and in 1963, almost two decades after the streptomycin investigation, he wrote: "In a controlled trial, as in all experimental work, there is no need in the search for precision to throw common sense out of the window."[30] After overcoming such problems, at the study's end in 1948 the investigators could declare that active tuberculosis "can be halted by streptomycin."[31]

When using historical controls and other common research techniques, investigators experienced difficulty in deciding if the effects witnessed were caused by the treatment, the natural course of the disease, the peculiarities of patients, their environments, or other extraneous factors. The controlled trial as it developed after 1948 and was refined sought to avoid these confusions through two essential features. First, it assembled similar groups of patients treated similarly except in a critical dimension: each group received different but look-alike treatments, one of which was the therapy being tested and the other one a control whose effects were already known – either a standard treatment or if one didn't exist or was ineffective a substance with no active ingredients, a placebo. Second, the study groups were formed through procedures that produced random assignments, for example, creating groups linked to the random generation of odd and even numbers, and that concealed the allocation schedule from participants. This helped eliminate selection bias. Another key aspect of controlled trials was the double-blind feature, in which neither the treatment team nor the patient knew which therapy the patient received. This was a further attempt to prevent the introduction of conscious or unconscious bias in the observations of those who conducted the study or the reports of those who received the therapy. The innovation that emerged, the double-blind, randomized controlled trial (RCT), came to be the gold standard of clinical investigations.

The streptomycin investigation deserves its status as a landmark randomized clinical trial not because it was the first, but for its innovative method to shield the allocation schedule from participants, as Chalmers points out, and for the attention it commanded in the medical world by the significance of its proof that a major new drug worked. Landmark efforts, as noted previously (see Chapter 3), need not be first efforts, but they can be ones that synthesize knowledge, demonstrate significance, and galvanize attention.

In the more than sixty years since the streptomycin trial occurred, some 1 million RCTs probably have been conducted. To maximize the knowledge of the RCT method, acclaimed as "the study design conferring the best evidence for effects of interventions," efforts began in the 1980s to identify a way of combining the results of multiple RCT studies, known as systemic reviews.[32] The need for such a synthesis of research findings was suggested most notably by the British researcher Archie Cochrane in his 1972 book *Effectiveness and Efficiency*, and first carried out on a large scale at a center named for him at Oxford University, founded in 1992. Such research synthesis is an endeavor to locate all the RCTs associated with a given issue. Once accomplished, the finding of different outcomes in studies asking the same question requires the development of criteria to winnow poorly conducted from well conducted studies, and to select from those the ones to be used to create the research synthesis.[33]

Systematic research reviews of RCTs are considered the best evidence of a therapy's effectiveness, superior to any single RCT. But in 2003 the movement drew attention to the absence of a system for registering all RCTs and disseminating their results, a problem since many of those conducted are never published and thus lost to scientific use.[34] Research into the reasons for not publishing RCTs found that investigators are influenced by favorable study results and lose interest in studies that produce negative findings.[35] If published RCTs were skewed in favor of those reporting positive findings about evaluated treatments, and thereby threatened the integrity of the research reviews of RCTs, significant efforts to right the balance seemed essential. Action was taken in the following year, when the International Committee of Medical Journal Editors, a group whose members included medicine's most prestigious journals, announced that, beginning in 2005, it would consider for publication only those clinical trials registered before they recruited their first patient, a requirement with a comprehensive and publicly accessible database of trials as their goal.[36] The editors urged other journals and governments to support the effort and declared: "A complete registry of trials would be a fitting way to thank the thousands of participants who have placed themselves at risk by volunteering for clinical trials. They deserve to prove that the information that accrues from their altruism is part of the public record, where it is available to guide decisions about patient care, and deserve to know that decisions about their care rest on all of the evidence, not just the trials authors decided to report and that journal editors decided to publish."[37]

But, establishing the scientific effectiveness of a technology influences only in part how it will be used. For example, relatively ineffective technologies that offer the only option in troubling or life-threatening illness are often requested by patients, applied by doctors, and paid for by insurance companies. To demonstrate how the joining of social values and scientific evidence determines the way technologies are used, and the emerging role of consumers in shaping this process, we turn to the remarkable interaction of the public, professional, and governmental communities who developed and implemented a plan to ration medical care in Oregon.

The Oregon story starts in 1987, when the state legislature voted to change the way it expended resources for Medicaid, a national program to provide health care to indigent people that federal and state governments jointly fund and states administer. Among other things, Oregon legislators concluded that the cost of organ transplantation was disproportionate to its low success rate and reallocated the transplant funds to support prenatal care for pregnant women and basic health care for children. But controversy arose when two patients were denied transplants because of the funding cuts. One of the families was forced to move to another state to secure an organ for an infant. The other case involved a seven-year-old boy with leukemia who died while his family was in the midst of a campaign to raise $100,000 to cover the cost of a bone-marrow transplant. His death spawned widespread media coverage and led citizen committees, advocacy groups, and the state legislature to confront the dilemma of how to allocate limited resources to an expanding array of medical therapies. The outcome was the passage of the 1989 Oregon Basic Health Services Act.

The reform rested on a bold decision to expand the number of people covered by state insurance and had three parts. First, a high-risk insurance pool was established to sell state-subsidized insurance to people whose preexisting health conditions made purchasing private-sector insurance impossible. Second, all employers would be required to provide health-care insurance to employees and their dependents by 1995 and given tax credits to help pay for it. The legislature mandated that the benefit package for the employer and high-risk coverage programs must be at least equivalent to the one designed for those on Medicaid, the changes to which were the most provocative element and centerpiece of the act.

This third portion of the reform expanded the number of indigent Oregonians covered by insurance by making all people with an income below the federal poverty level (at the time about $900 per month for a family of three) eligible for Medicaid. But the expansion was possible only by reducing the costs per covered person in the new plan. And the controversial step proposed to accomplish this was limiting provided health services to those deemed to have the greatest impact on securing beneficial medical outcomes. To accomplish this, Oregon established a public- and expert-based process through which therapies made available to the Medicaid population would be chosen. Such an effort on this scale had never been made before. And this novelty brought the federal government into the picture. Since it dispensed matching funds to states under the Medicaid program, implementation of the Oregon plan required a number of federal regulations to be waived. As a result, the high-profile public dialogue in Oregon about the benefits the plan should provide, and the congressional debate about whether to approve it, made the plan a lightning rod of national discussion and controversy.[38]

As the arm to reform Medicaid in Oregon, the 1989 act created a Health Services Commission, whose eleven members included five physicians, four consumers, a nurse, and a social worker. Its main task was developing a list that prioritized the value of various health interventions. The list and estimates of the cost of funding each of its interventions would be given to the governor and legislature to determine the package of benefits offered to recipients of Oregon's Medicaid program, and thereby set not only its budget but also the budgets of the high-risk pool and employer insurance programs, which used the Medicaid benefit package as their norm.

The Oregon approach embodied three ethical ideals: it is more just to provide a reduced but more effective basket of health benefits to a wider population than a greater but less beneficial basket of benefits to a smaller number of people; publicly accountable and openly made rationing choices were preferable to ones that, in the current system, were hidden from view; and community opinions and expert judgments should be merged to create health priorities in the state.[39]

The commission used cost-effectiveness analysis to generate an initial list of prioritized services. In this method, based on the principle of gaining the greatest benefit for the most people, an effective life-sustaining therapy could be downgraded by its high cost or the fact that it benefited few people, and so fall toward the bottom of the list. In May 1990, applying a cost-effectiveness formula, the commission developed a list having this character. Thus, its first almost one hundred items were for conditions usually treatable in a doctor's office, while a significant ailment needing hospital care could receive a relatively low rating because of its higher cost.[40] Negative public reaction to this approach led the commission to generate a new priority list using a ranking method focused less on cost and more on a therapy's value to individuals, to the community, and to improving quality of life.

To create this list, a two-part strategy was developed. In one part, thousands of Oregonians spread across geographic, ethnic, and income lines were surveyed by telephone and convened in public meetings to explore their views about the effects of illness on daily life; the benefits, burdens, and economic cost of alternative treatments; and the health services they valued most. To focus discourse at the public meetings participants were presented with brief scenarios and asked to discuss the provision of therapy under the circumstances outlined in them. Here is one: "After three heart attacks, a patient is getting worse despite taking several medications daily. An operation to put in a pacemaker would probably help the heart's rhythm but not the general condition of the heart. The day to day activities of the patient may improve" (see Table 1).[41] In the other part of the strategy, commission members – informed by the public opinion data, the work of groups of Oregon medical experts, and ideas in the health literature – developed a priority list of 709 treatments, each linked to particular medical conditions such as appendicitis. The criteria they used included, among others, how a given treatment influenced the quality of life of affected individuals, the treatment's value to society, and its significance within a basic package of health benefits.[42]

In May 1991 the commission submitted its suggestions on ones to fund to the state legislature, which decided to support most of the therapies down to No. 587 of the 709-item list, approving with few exceptions the commission's recommendations (see Table 2). The list of funded therapies favored preventive services, treatments helping women and children, and those that restored the health of affected patients. Treatments for acute conditions were selected over those for chronic ones. Cost was not a prominent factor in determining rank; indeed, more than half the treatments having high costs were placed in the top half of the list. The list's rankings also emphasized social over individual need; thus, treatments that were characterized as "valuable to certain individuals" received the lowest-priority ratings on the list, and very few of them were funded. As the commission noted in its report to the legislature: "What is essential for the overall well-being of the society may not meet the desires of specific individuals. Responding to the needs of both society and the individual may mean earmarking more funds for investment in Oregon's medical assistance programs than has previously been the case."[43]

Reactions to the Oregon rationing proposal were mixed. It was criticized as a flawed document for a faulty analysis of treatment benefits that damaged the validity of the prioritized list;[44] for its inadequate attention to the justice principle, which required not only explicit

TABLE I. *Health-care values elicited at community meetings. Office of Technology Assessment. Evaluation of the Oregon Medicaid Proposal. (OTA-H-531) U.S. Government Printing Office, May 1992, 49.*

- Prevention – Preventive services such as prenatal care and childhood immunizations were unanimously agreed upon as essential.
- Quality of life – Services that enhance emotional and physical well-being, as well as extend life, were generally thought to increase quality of life and should receive higher priority than those that only extend life.
- Cost effectiveness – Cost-effective treatments were given high priority, although some community members disagreed that cost alone should be a primary determinant in prioritization.
- Ability to function – The importance of independence and ability to perform daily activities was mentioned at three-fourths of the community meetings.
- Equity – Equity was described as a fundamental belief that everyone should have equal access to adequate health care. Discussions of equity raised various objections to the prioritization process – many participants, for instance, thought that health care services should be available equally to all segments of society. There *was* support for increased Federal funding for health care services, and some advocated the establishment of a national health insurance plan. Other equity issues discussed included increasing access to treatment services in rural communities and universal access to health care for children.
- Effectiveness of treatment – Participants agreed that treatments with proven efficacy and those that improve quality of life should be prioritized over those less likely to have successful outcomes.
- Benefits many – Services that benefit many should receive higher priority than those for whom few benefit, according to participants.
- Mental health and chemical dependency – Prevention, including drug education, was more highly valued than treatment services. While mental health and chemical dependency services were frequently discussed at meetings, there was some ambivalence regarding society's obligation to provide substance abuse services. Some participants, for example, felt that treatment was appropriate only in cases where patients were "motivated to undergo treatment," and that recidivism needed to be considered in cases of "repeat offenders."
- Personal choice – Some community members expressed a desire for increased choice of type of providers, while others wanted more patient and family autonomy in making medical treatment decisions.
- Community compassion – Participants indicated that society is obligated to provide treatments and services that alleviate pain and suffering (e.g., hospice care).
- Impact on society – Treatments for infectious diseases and for alcoholism or drug abuse are examples of services that yield societal as well as individual benefit (discussed at approximately half of the community meetings).
- Length of life – Prolonging life was viewed as important, but a treatment's value is limited if extending life sacrifices quality of life.
- Personal responsibility – Personal responsibility was viewed as the individual's obligation to society to seek appropriate health education and treatment services, and to generally take responsibility for one's health. Individuals taking responsibility for their health should receive priority, and those whose illnesses are related to lifestyle, such as alcohol- and drug-related conditions, a low priority if health care services are rationed.

Source: R. Hasnain and M. Garland, "Health Care in Common: Report of the Oregon Health Decisions Community Meetings Process," Oregon Health Decisions, Portland, OR, April 1990.

TABLE 2. *The seventeen services categories used in the prioritization process. The 709 conditions developed through the commission's work were classified into seventeen categories, which in turn were grouped under three headings indicating how the commission valued the health services within them. The Oregon Legislature, largely following the commission's recommendations, funded all services described as "essential," all but eight of the services described as "very important;" and only five of those described as "valuable to certain individuals." Office of Technology Assessment. Evaluation of the Oregon Medicaid Proposal (OTA-H-531). U.S. Government Printing Office, May 1992, 47.*

Category	Description
"Essential" services	
1. Acute fatal	Treatment prevents death with full recovery. *Example: Appendectomy for appendicitis.*
2. Maternity care	Maternity and most newborn care. *Example: Obstetrical care for pregnancy.*
3. Acute fatal	Treatment prevents death without full recovery. *Example: Medical therapy for acute bacterial meningitis.*
4. Preventive care for children	*Example: Immunizations.*
5. Chronic fatal	Treatment improves life span and quality of life. *Example: Medical therapy for asthma.*
6. Reproductive services	Excludes maternity/infertility services. *Example: Contraceptive management.*
7. Comfort care	Palliative therapy for conditions in which death is imminent. *Example: Hospice care.*
8. Preventive dental care	Adults and children. *Example: Cleaning and fluoride applications.*
9. Proven effective preventive care for adults	*Example: Mammograms.*
"Very important" services	
10. Acute nonfatal	Treatment causes return to previous health state. *Example: Medical therapy for vaginitis.*
11. Chronic nonfatal	One-time treatment improves quality of life. *Example: Hip replacement.*
12. Acute nonfatal	Treatment without return to previous health state. *Example: Arthroscopic repair of internal knee derangement.*
13. Chronic nonfatal	Repetitive treatment improves quality of life. *Example: Medical therapy for chronic sinusitis.*
Services that are "valuable to certain individuals"	
14. Acute nonfatal	Treatment expedites recovery of self-limiting conditions. *Example: Medical therapy for diaper rash.*
15. Infertility services	*Example: In-vitro fertilization.*
16. Less effective preventive care for adults	*Example: Screening of nonpregnant adults for diabetes.*
17. Fatal or nonfatal	Treatment causes minimal or no improvement in quality of life. *Example: Medical therapy for viral warts.*

Source: Oregon Health Services Commission Salem, OR, "Prioritized Health Services List," May 1, 1991.

consideration of the total quantity of benefits produced by its plan but also the morality of how the benefits were distributed among potential claimants;[45] for extending Medicaid coverage to new beneficiaries who were mainly single adults and childless couples by reducing benefits (via the cutoff point on the priority list) for the about one hundred thousand current Medicaid beneficiaries, most of whom were Oregon's poorest women of childbearing age and their children;[46] for its use of quality of life indices to construct its priority rankings, flawed by dependence on third parties to judge the meaning of a life, a view that only those affected by the illness could authentically give;[47] for the use of a state rationing approach as a substitute for a comprehensive national health plan that would equitably care for all segments of society;[48] and for being a rationing plan selectively aimed at the poor rather than the whole population of Oregon.[49]

The Oregon plan also was lauded for the candor of a legislature publicly admitting it could not give unlimited health-care access to all and explicitly indicating how it would ration resources;[50] for protecting poor people by locking in health benefits for them;[51] for achieving a dramatic change in the way its citizens gained health care that was generally accepted by them and expanding health coverage to all poor Oregonians;[52] and for the possibility of demonstrating a means of containing costs through a priority system that could model a future effort to achieving universal health care in the United States.[53]

Using procedures such as controlled clinical trials to reduce the effect of the convictions and hopes of involved investigators and subjects in generating and interpreting experimental findings has produced dependable evidence about the biological effectiveness of contemporary therapies. Complementing this knowledge is the growth of quantitative techniques to evaluate therapies in terms of nonbiological benefits, such as lengthening the years and quality of life and minimizing the monetary cost of doing so. Taken together, the procedures provide a foundation upon which to decide how to allocate therapeutic resources.

But Oregon complemented the two forms of analysis with a third and innovative category. It created a statewide public dialogue about distributing health resources that focused on ethical values, social needs, funding limits, and the meaning and effects of therapies on daily living – allied to a commission having a broad public and professional composition to interpret and merge the public perspective with its own views in formulating recommendations to the state legislature. By these steps, Oregon added a public voice to the choir of clinical and socioeconomic evidence that usually dominates resource allocation in medicine, which made the evidence more compelling to hear and follow.

AMID THE TECHNOLOGICAL TRIUMPHS OF DISEASE PREVENTION

Where Is Health?

Nineteen seventeen is famous as the year when the United States entered the First World War. It also is infamous in medical circles for a related event – as the time when the nation learned the results of its first national physical examination. Before they could enter the fighting force, the millions of individuals drafted or inspired to volunteer for service first had to pass through a medical screen of doctors and technology. The results were totally unexpected – and disastrous. Some 550,000 of the approximately 3.8 million recruits between the ages of eighteen and forty-two examined were rejected as unfit for military service. And to make matters worse, of the about 2.7 million who eventually entered the armed forces, almost half had physical impairments.

To find 15 percent of a population thought to be in the prime of life too unhealthy to fight for their country was a devastating blow to national pride and a shock to the nation's doctors. It was widely labeled in medical journals "the horrible example."[1] If this weren't bad enough, two other factors made matters worse. A large number of the conditions that led to rejection for service were preventable or treatable, such as vision defects, tuberculosis, venereal diseases, and foot problems. Further, if such widespread disease and disability were prevalent in the part of the American population believed to be the most healthy, it seemed reasonable to expect a worse result when the true condition of the segments who were younger or older were studied. Now, almost a century later, we continue to grapple with the issues of the scale on which we should look for hidden disease, what to do with ambiguous results the search can generate, and how to define disease and attain the elusive state called health.

Exploration of these issues requires an understanding of how health and illness are treated in the two major but opposing theories that sequentially have guided thought and action in Western medicine over the past 2,500 years. One, the environmentalist concept, examined and described most fully in ancient Greece, proposed health and illness to be transitory states resulting from the changing interactions of individuals and the environments in which they live and by which they are enveloped. A second, the structuralist concept, had its origin about four hundred years ago during the Renaissance. It proposed that diseases were tangible realities linked to structural changes in parts of the body that could alter normal function and that health was a state in which the body was free of such defects. The effects of these theories will be explored here.

In Greece during the fifth century BCE, an environmentalist approach to health and illness was created that had a remarkable run of more than two millennia as the conceptual basis of medicine before relinquishing its reign in the nineteenth century. It was led by a figure whose work remains vital and read to this day, and whose name is synonymous with the highest ideals of medicine – Hippocrates. He founded a school of medicine that generated important works for several centuries. He was born on the island of Kos and traveled widely about the Greek archipelago. He was long-lived and honored as the greatest physician of his day. Little more is known about his life.

But much is known about his views and those of his disciples. They are proclaimed in extensive writings, which include significant commentaries on a concept of health and illness upon which the medicine of his time was developed and practiced – the humoral theory, briefly touched on in the previous chapter. It declared that the basic components and life forces of the body were fluid substances called humors. Four in number, they were described as blood, phlegm, black bile, and yellow bile. Balance and proportionality were the central facts of their biological relationship. The greatest state of health occurred when the humors were in a stable equilibrium, which meant that the proportion of each humor to the others was ideal. When one or more humors became enlarged or diminished, the stability of the equilibrium was damaged and disability or illness ensued. Thus, the role of the doctor was to prescribe actions that patients could take to maintain a stability within their biological selves, producing the harmony of health and preventing the discord of illness. And when illness occurred, the doctor's job was to identify the discordant humor and initiate therapies that rebalanced the humor and restored stability. What gives this theory its significance is explaining health and illness through a unitary concept and assigning equal standing to each.

To go along with a concept of how the body functioned to produce the states of health and illness, there remained an equally important matter for the Greeks to clarify – explaining what led to humoral dysfunction. Here they developed a far-reaching and profound view of disease causation. The Greeks discerned two basic environments within and through which humans functioned. One was the just-considered internal biological sphere, whose most essential aspect was the interplay of its humoral components. A second was an external worldly sphere most crucially influenced by mode of life – what people ate and drank, whether they exercised and rested appropriately, their mental composure and response to the mores and customs that bound them to society – and by the natural world they inhabited, its soil and waters, climate and seasons, winds and elevation. Stimuli from this external sphere influenced internal humoral function and relationships, disruptively to cause illness or accommodatively to maintain humoral balance and health.

The linkage of the external environment to health and illness is innovatively, wisely, and elegantly portrayed in the Hippocratic work *Airs, Waters, Places*. It advises physicians entering a new city "to consider its situation, how it lies as to the winds and the rising of the sun . . . whether it be naked and deficient in water, or wooded and well watered, and whether it lies in a hollow, confined situation, or is elevated and cold; and the mode in which the inhabitants live, and what are their pursuits, whether they are fond of drinking and eating to excess, and given to indolence, or are fond of exercise and labour, and not given to excess in eating and drinking." If the doctor worked hard to acquire these facts and from them discerned the illnesses peculiar to and common in these places, he would not make mistakes in his treatments and would be able to predict "what epidemic diseases will attack the city, either in summer or in winter, and what each individual will be in danger of experiencing from the change of regimen. For knowing the changes of the seasons, the risings and settings of the stars, how each of them takes place, he will be able to know beforehand what sort of a year is going to ensue. Having made these investigations, and knowing beforehand the seasons, such a one... must succeed in the preservation of health, and be by no means unsuccessful in the practice of his art."[2]

Airs, Waters, Places is possibly the most cogently titled scientific treatise on health, illness, and the environment. It also is a seminal work, providing the first theoretical and practical perspective on why understanding illness and prescribing actions to secure and enhance health in individuals necessitated a perspective on where and how they lived. Since most Greek doctors needed to travel among the towns and islands of Greece to make a living, an ability to analyze the natural settings and lifestyles of the new places they encountered was crucial to their ability to succeed as healers.

But in addition to this environmental perspective, another matter influenced the ability of Greek doctors to be successful. It is announced in the opening line of another significant but brief Hippocratic essay, "The Physician," which outlines the basis of an ethical medical life: "The dignity of a physician requires that he should look healthy, and as plump as nature intended him to be; for the common crowd consider those who are not of this excellent bodily condition to be unable to take care of others."[3] It was not enough for Greek doctors to support the ideal of seeking health through sound choices of living but to act on it. How could patients trust the advice of doctors who from their appearance seemed uncommitted to their proclaimed beliefs? As to the association in this document of plumpness with health, modest corpulence in individuals was a sign that they did not suffer from the wasting illnesses prevalent in ancient Greece.

In summary, the idea of balance – among the basic constituents of the self, and of the self with the essential elements of the natural and social world – was the foundation of treating illness and preserving health and the essence of the environmentalist concept. But now we examine the view that followed and replaced the environmentalist perspective as the conceptual underpinning of medicine, the structuralist concept.

Two basic lines of thought converge to develop this perspective. One is that diseases are things – unitary, tangible objects whose unique constellations of effects distinguish one from another. A second is that these things take up residence and leave traces in body structures that are both signatures of their identity and causes of disordered function.

The idea that diseases are distinct objects was most fully developed in the seventeenth century by an English physician who also carried the name of Hippocrates but as a mantle of honor. Thomas Sydenham, dubbed "the English Hippocrates" to acknowledge his extraordinary ability to detect and recognize the significance of clinical symptoms felt and displayed by patients, studied and practiced medicine in an age devoted to exploring the natural world to identify and categorize its plants and animals. Scholars traveled the globe for this purpose and published the results of their efforts in herbals, manuscripts, and printed books that illustrated plants and described their medicinal characteristics. Their work influenced Sydenham, as did his study of the Hippocratic writings, with their emphases on careful observation of the effects of illness on individuals, and the views of the seventeenth-century scientist and philosopher Francis Bacon on defining groups on the basis of the similarity of their constituents.

But the reigning concept of health and illness, the humoral theory, generally did not distinguish and name particular illnesses or have specific remedies for them. Instead, it created general categories of sickness such as whole-body disorders (fevers) and dysfunctions in body organs such as the intestines (dysenteries), lungs (pleurisies), eyes (ophthalmies), and so forth, the outcomes of humoral imbalance. After determining that the humors were out of balance, physicians practiced a medicine grounded in prognosis, an effort to predict how the disorder would develop given the symptoms felt by the patient and signs of bodily dysfunction observed by the doctor. The goal of the therapy developed from these projections was also general, to restore humoral order, with treatment modified on a regular basis as the course of the illness played out. Such a method did not necessitate naming disorders, the general exceptions being epidemic illness in which many people had a similar set of symptoms and suffered a similar outcome, and sickness with unique symptoms such as epilepsy.

Prognostic medicine practiced at its best demands rapt attention to changes in the character and course of a patient's symptoms, thus making a doctor's ability to observe them and glean their present and future meaning the mark of medical excellence. Sydenham was gifted in this respect, which allowed him to transform the generic perspective of doctors toward illness. His extraordinary talent in clinical observation and intellectual vision converged to produce this great insight: illnesses, like plants and creatures of the natural world, were true entities that received an identity through tangible features; just as a plant's universal characteristics applied to all members of its species, likewise the symptoms of a disease were expressed in those who carried it. Sydenham wrote: "Nature, in the production of disease, is uniform and consistent; so much so, that for the same disease in different persons the symptoms are for the most part the same, and the self same phenomenon that you would observe in the sickness of a Socrates you would observe in the sickness of a simpleton."[4] And from Sydenham's conclusion that diseases, like plants, could be described and classified like other entities of the natural world, followed the insight that specific remedies could be discovered to treat those specific diseases, a view affirmed in the success he had in treating a defined illness, malaria, with a particular remedy, quinine.

The method Sydenham used to distinguish diseases was creative and demanding. He divided the symptoms of illness into two categories – those that were unique expressions of the individual experiencing the sickness and those that were definitive elements of the malady shared by all who had it. To make this distinction in even one disorder required an extraordinary perceptive skill; applied to observing numerous patients over time to identify the many ailments he uncovered was a tour de force. For the basic symptoms of the disease entities he described needed to be sequenced into a pattern having a beginning, middle, and end, which included the context within which they typically occurred and other characteristics that would clearly distinguish one disease from another, particularly when the symptoms of different entities were similar. Not only did Sydenham define new diseases; he also described disorders that had already been recognized as distinct but that, from lack of a clear analysis of their nature, caused doctors to miss or confuse them with others. Here are two examples of the portraits of disease drawn by Sydenham. The first depicts what we now call tuberculosis but then was called phthisis, and the second is measles.

Phthisis

The cough betrays itself. The phthisis comes on between the eighteenth and thirty-fifth years. The whole body becomes emaciated. There is a troublesome, hectic cough which is increased by taking food and which is distinguished by the quickness of the pulse, and the redness of the cheeks. The matter spit up by the cough is bloody or purulent. When burnt it smells fetid. When thrown into water it sinks. Night sweats supervene. At length the cheeks grow hard, the face pale, the nose sharp. The temples sink, the nails curve inward, the hair falls off, there is colloquitative diarrhoea, the forerunner of death.

Measles

The measles generally attack children. On the first day they have chills and shivers, and are hot and cold in turns. On the second they have the fever in full – disquietude, thirst, want of appetite, a white (but not a dry) tongue, slight cough, heaviness of the head and eyes, and somnolence. The nose and eyes run continuously; and this is the surest sign of measles. The symptoms increase till the fourth day. Then – or sometimes on the fifth – there appear on the face and forehead small red spots, very like the bites of fleas. These increase in number, and cluster together, so as to mark the face with large red blotches.

The spots take hold of the face first; from which they spread to the chest and belly, and afterwards to the legs and ankles. There is slight cough, which, with the fever and the difficulty of breathing, increases. There is also a running from the eyes. On the sixth day, or thereabout, the forehead and face begin to grow rough, as the pustules die off, and the skin breaks. About the eighth day they disappear from the face, and scarcely show on the rest of the body. On the ninth, there are none anywhere.[5]

With the acute senses and human insight of a great clinical artist, Sydenham drew these stunningly authentic portraits of disease, a medical Cervantes who shared with his Spanish contemporary a genius for literary depiction and empathy. Indeed, it would be hard to write a better introductory line for phthisis than "the cough betrays itself." We learn when the disease appears, how it is announced, the matter it generates, and the reaction of this substance to heat and liquid. The sequence of body responses to the ailment is given with a succinct and progressive gravity, concluding with a sign that foretells the end.

In his account of measles, Sydenham begins by pinpointing its main target – children. Since measles is usually an acute, short-term disorder, he provides a concise account of its day-to-day expression: the temperature shifts of day one, the barrage of body responses to the attack in the next four, including a single constant that was the disorder's "surest sign," unstoppable runny nose and eyes. Thus, even before the most dramatic aspect of the disease appears – the measles themselves – a diagnosis is possible. When the red spots come, likened whimsically but accurately to bites of the flea, Sydenham describes their change of appearance and sequence of attack much like a military officer's precise account of a battle, which ends after a nine-day seige with the enemy in full withdrawal.

By thus establishing illnesses as entities, Sydenham achieved his goal of connecting them with specific meliorating remedies. He also changed medicine fundamentally by gradually turning the doctor's role from the individually focused technique of prognosis to the group-centered discipline of diagnosis. For having named the entity making the patient sick made it possible to seek a standard therapy that worked and could be applied to all patients in this category.

But as we learned from the voyage of the stethoscope in the medical waters of the nineteenth century, great ideas may be overextended by enthusiastic adopters, and zealous embrace can prove as deadly as damning skepticism. Sydenham's concept of diseases as entities had its authenticity deeply tested by successors who, like those obsessed with conspiracy theories, saw disease in any place where two or more symptoms might meet. Most notable among these enthusiasts was François Bossier de Sauvages, a botanist and physician, who in 1763 published a large book titled *Nosologia methodica, sistems morborum classes, genera et species*. It declared the existence of some 2,400 diseases, which included itching, snoring, and hiccup. Fortunately, this work and others like it were effectively criticized by scholars who appreciated the reach and limit of disease classification and advanced the concept more judiciously.

As did his contemporaries, Sydenham continued to adhere to the humoral theory as the causal basis of illness and health. However, he modified its basic conceptual framework to fit his vision of disease. He proposed that environmental conditions led humors to "become exalted into a *substantial form* or *species*," and thereby generate specific diseases that reflected these changes.[6] Sydenham also considered the significance of a major line of new thinking, which focused on autopsy of the body and dissection as the basic means of learning about the nature of disease. He rejected anatomical study for this purpose on the grounds that it diverted medicine from a far more significant avenue to defining and understanding diseases – the discipline of clinical observation and the study of symptoms at the bedside. For Sydenham, this was the bedrock of medicine.

However, others thought differently. Influenced by the pioneering work of Andreas Vesalius, who studied normal anatomical structures in his 1543 work *De humani corporis fabrica*, contemporaries and successors of Sydenham saw in the autopsy a crucial path to learning how diseases developed and how their effects were caused. The central figure in this exploration of the human anatomical landscape was an Italian physician whom we have briefly met in an earlier chapter, Giovanni Battista Morgagni. His accomplishment was as signal as Sydenham's. He wove together several centuries of anatomical observations of normal and diseased bodies with his own large personal experience at the autopsy table to construct the masterwork that has defined the basic medical view of health and illness ever since: his 1761 treatise *The Seats and Causes of Diseases Investigated by Anatomy*.

The structure of this grand work is quite simple. It is divided into five sections, each of which considers a major region of the body, such as the head and the thorax, and the significant clinical disorders to which the region is prone. Each disorder in turn is analyzed through the presentation of case reports, which start with a description of how the illness evolved, followed by an account of the dissection after death and concluding with a commentary linking the structural defects revealed by autopsy with their clinical expressions in life. But the most significant feature is two sets of indices, the first of which

shows what has been observed in living bodies, the other what in the bodies after death; so that if any physician observe a singular, or any other symptoms in a patient, and desire to know what internal injury is wont to correspond to that symptom; or if any anatomist find any particular morbid appearance in the dissection of a body, and should wish to know what symptom has preceded an injury of this kind in other bodies; the physician, by inspecting the first of these indexes, the anatomist by inspecting the second, will immediately find the observation which contains both (if both have been observ'd by us).[7]

The indices summed up the benefits that the marriage of anatomic pathology and bedside medicine brought to studying and diagnosing disease, and thus assumed large practical and scientific value.

The significance of structural disorder in the body's fabric inevitably drew Morgagni into the issue of ultimate causation: what generated the lesions? Morgagni pointed out obvious causes such as heredity or accidental life circumstances. But he refused to be drawn into discussions about the ultimate sources of illness, "which man can under no circumstances attain."[8] He considered causal speculations fruitless diversions from studying how symptoms sprang from disordered anatomy and how this learning could be enlisted in the battle against illness.

Sydenham and Morgagni were the central figures in the consolidation and creation of knowledge that drastically changed medical thinking and practice. Sydenham mapped illness at the surface of life. He was an expert at navigating the rapids of the feelings and physical effects of illness, and at extracting from these currents the precious gems that revealed what was wrong. But the world of Morgagni had no swift currents. His was a world at repose. Their earthly days over, there remained engraved within the corpses he dissected evidence of what had been. For Morgagni, the physician-cum-archaeologist, the ultimate goal was the reconstruction of events leading the internal structures of the body to become what they were, and thus account for the turmoil at its surface that was the life symptoms of disease. And most critically, their individual work came together to support the transformative concept that illness was caused by tangible entities distinguished from one another by the marks they left both outside and within the body.

The structuralist concept of disease stormed nineteenth-century medicine, upending and supplanting humoralism as the theoretical basis of medicine. It was borne on a wave of technological innovation that breached the outer covering of the body and carried the physician into a living and revelatory inner terrain. The new technologies permitted doctors to capture the sounds of the body doing its work, to probe the composition of its fluids, to fathom the state of its biological systems, and most dramatically, to visually display its intricate landscape – a process that located hidden diseases and defined them with a new scientific precision.

Gradually, organ after organ gave up secrets of hidden workings to new technological probes, such as the stethoscope, ophthalmoscope, and X-ray; so, too, did crucial body functions like temperature and blood pressure, whose waxing and waning were followed precisely with quantitatively based technologies; likewise with crucial fluids like blood and pivotal wastes such as urine, whose components were analyzed and monitored by techniques and machines brought together to form medical laboratories. These findings, in turn, were tested by and correlated with structural changes in the body's fabric, a process that itself was advanced dramatically by technological improvements in the microscope.

Using this instrument, the German physician Rudolf Virchow developed the findings for his 1858 landmark work *Cellular Pathology*. It portrayed the body as a cellular state and advanced the view that while current and future research had and would discover biological elements smaller than the cell, it was and would remain the most fundamental expression of biological existence. As Morgagni had demonstrated on the organs and surrounding structures of the body characteristic footprints left on them by diseases, so Virchow did on the body's cells. Virchow thus redefined health and illness on the basis of anatomical and functional changes in cells. And as did Morgagni, Virchow affirmed that diseases had seats in the body revealed through specific changes in its architecture. He wrote: "No physician can properly think out a process of disease unless he is able to fix for it a place in the body." To Virchow, the chief question for physicians and scientists probing the human frame to heal and learn from it was "*Ubi est morbus?* Where is the disease?"[9]

While Morgagni and Virchow convincingly demonstrated the nature and sites of the where-is-the-disease issue, in 1882 an extraordinary scientific paper addressed the what-is-disease puzzle. And the answer reaffirmed the concept of diseases as unique and concrete entities. The bombshell was dropped on the world's medical community by the German physician Robert Koch when he announced: "For the first time, the parasitic nature of a human infective disease, and, indeed, of the most important of all diseases, has been completely demonstrated."[10] Koch had discovered the bacterial agent that caused tuberculosis, then responsible for the deaths of approximately one in seven individuals in the Europe of the nineteenth century. Further, and in a comprehensive way that set a scientific standard for such investigations, this proof opened the door to a vast inquiry into the role of bacteria in other human afflictions. And as this line of research flourished, it generated a hope that identifying the bacterial sources of illness was the first step in the emergence of an era in which the conquest of disease was possible.

Into this climate a new concept – the periodic medical examination – burst onto the scene with the mission of evaluating the general condition of people and turning American medicine into a disease-preventing, health-creating discipline. Enthusiasm for it was generated by a confluence of technological advances and social needs, which began with doctors seeking to maximize the potential of their technology to detect the presence of disease in stages so early that victims were unaware of its lurking presence. The possibility of early detection improved the chances both of the patient's recovery and, if the disorder was contagious, of preventing its spread to others. The concept interested schools, industry, and the public, which led them to use the periodic examination in a host of ways and make it a central vehicle in the quest for a healthy America.

In its early phases, the periodic examination focused on audiences controlled by organizations. Over time, its medical scope was broadened and its social reach extended to assess individuals. Schools were its first users, influenced by the massive influx of immigrants into the United States at the turn of the twentieth century. The poverty of immigrant children made them vulnerable to illnesses, which endangered the health of the American-born children whom they learned with in schools – a situation made worse in major cities where immigrants were a majority of pupils. This linked the health and welfare of the country to the health and welfare of its schools. As Lillian Wald, a leading social reformer of this period, put it: "Education should aim to develop good minds, good habits, good characters, good citizens, and this cannot be accomplished unless the mental training and the methods of education are directly influenced by the physical life and constitution of the individual child."[11]

The medical survey of schoolchildren in America started in the late nineteenth century as a means to detect contagious illness, but it soon expanded to cover other areas such as sight. Studies in 1905 found vision poor enough to limit learning in a third to a fifth of examined students.[12] S. Josephine Baker, a physician who evaluated school children for New York City at about this time, found widespread disabilities as well as a disturbing level of infectious disorders in them. Some 80 percent had head lice, and contagious skin disorders such as ringworm, impetigo, and scabies were pervasive. She likened the schoolrooms to "contagious disease wards with all the different diseases so mingled it was a wonder that each child did not have all of them." Yet the general examination produced moments of hilarity, often erupting at Baker's initial physical inspection: "When I entered the room the children all arranged themselves in a line and passed before me in solemn procession, each child stopping for a moment, opening his mouth hideously wide and pulling down his lower eyelids with his fingers. For the children's purposes it was a beautiful opportunity for making a face at teacher unscathed and they made the most of it." The examinations and the interventions they generated greatly helped the children. For example, those with contagious diseases were treated and kept away from classes until the infection ended. And measures to prevent illness through disease testing and vaccination were initiated, such as one in New York City against diphtheria in the 1920s, which immunized almost three hundred thousand children and in one year alone (1928) helped drive down the disorder's death rate by a third.[13]

Intrigued by its benefits, industries followed schools in embracing periodic examinations. They helped companies hire workers best suited to perform particular jobs, prevented the spread of infectious disease within the workplace, and thus improved industrial production and efficiency. By the mid-1910s more than 10 percent of the three hundred largest corporations in the United States used the examinations to select and monitor worker health. A prominent medical journal extolled their promise: "If universally adopted, it would mean a physically and mentally better country. The sinews of production ever strengthened and guarded, the factory would cease to be considered a consumer of human lives, but would be considered rather an educator and supervisor of health."[14]

But the concept was controversial. Unions worried that the data employers accumulated about worker health could be shared among members of an industry and used to create a blacklist of those labeled as unfit. The access of employers to personal information about their workers also raised privacy and civil liberties concerns. In this debate about the distribution and use of personal health data, we see the antecedents of the confidentiality-of-patient-information problem in the health care of today.

Despite these problems, the concept of periodic examination spread beyond schools and factories to attract the attention of the public. An important organization in this effort was the Life Extension Institute, founded in 1914. It hired general practitioners to provide annual checkups to individuals and to businesses like insurance companies, and in its first decade conducted more than 250,000 examinations. The institute also performed a significant public service by educating the several thousand generalist physicians hired to do this work in the ideology and practice of preventive medicine, which had changed as the decade of the 1910s ended. This was reflected in the evolution of the periodic examination, which was broadened from its initial goal of uncovering hidden illness to also identifying habits of life that endangered health. Indeed, the movement's leaders believed that changes in lifestyle, then called hygiene, implemented through the periodic examination had become more important to public health than sanitary engineering projects geared to overcome environmental dangers such as the spread of infectious disease. The rationale for this judgment was a decline in communicable illnesses and a rise in the prevalence of chronic diseases such as cancer and disorders of the heart and kidneys. To influence the course of the latter type of illness required early diagnosis, education, and preventive habits of living – the sorts of interventions provided by the periodic checkup.[15] But no event more tellingly demonstrated its significance than the first physical examination of the American population, which evaluated the health of would-be soldiers for the First World War.

As mentioned at the chapter's beginning, gauging the fitness of recruits thought most able to fight for their country produced surprising and devastating results. It disclosed considerable disability and disease, which not only led to a rejection rate of nearly one in six but also found mostly disorders they could have prevented or treated. "The horrible example," as this outcome was dubbed, catalyzed the search to discover infirmities in other segments of the population when the war ended. The findings were as bad as feared: disorders identified in a sample of workers, 100 percent; immigrants, 97 percent; the general public, 77 percent. Some of the infirmities were not disabling, and the severity of others turned on the problem of defining normality.[16] But these results inspired advocates of the periodic examination to impress its value upon the public.

In the 1920s they did so aggressively, garnering support for annual examinations from health departments, the military, industrial corporations, and medical organizations. These groups bombarded the public with ad campaigns urging them to visit a doctor for an annual checkup. "Have a Health Examination on Your Birthday" was the banner under which the National Health Council launched a 1923 campaign to get 10 million Americans checked up.[17] At about this time a poster appeared in New York City subway cars proclaiming: "Your body is a wonderful machine. You own and operate it. You can't buy new lungs and a heart when your own are worn out. Let a doctor overhaul you once a year."[18] The metaphor of the body as a machine that needed regular upkeep drew upon the public love affair with the automobile, whose effective operation called for routine maintenance. Was the need for annual checkups to keep the human body running right any different? advocates of annual exams asked the car-loving nation.

Further proof of the substandard health of the population came in the mid-1930s, when the National Health Survey discovered one or more chronic illnesses in some 25 million Americans. In the early 1940s the Second World War attached an exclamation point to these findings. Determining the ability of recruits to fight spawned a second national medical examination, this time of some 20 million people. Its result was more dismal than the first one. A third of those examined were declared unfit to serve for physical and mental reasons. During and immediately after the war, periodic examination again was looked to by the public, medical profession, and government as a crucial means to discover, treat, and prevent illness.

In the 1950s, however, signs abounded that the periodic examination orchestrated and led by physicians was not the basic answer to the national problem of preventing illness and achieving health. The popularity of annual and often mandated examination of schoolchildren was waning and the Life Extension Institute, the early advocate and national sponsor of periodic examinations, discontinued this work. To make things worse, a new application of the concept, an elaborate and expensive annual examination for executives and the wealthy, was criticized as exemplifying the disparity of preventive interventions for the rich and the poor. But other indications of the examination's limits had been apparent since its origin. The intensive ad campaigns in the 1920s did not draw large numbers of people into doctors' offices. Indeed, since its introduction, the main constituents for the examination remained organizations – insurance companies, industries, schools, the military, and the like – not individuals.

The main reason for this outcome was neither social nor economic but conceptual. The periodic examination had elements of the doctor's usual general checkup, which featured a brief conversation about how the patient felt, listening with the stethoscope to tune in the heart and lungs, taking the temperature, and measuring the blood pressure. It differed by focusing more on physical evaluations like testing hearing and vision, but most critical and distinct was the viewpoint on which the periodic examination was based. Its goal was to appraise the life of patients to learn and influence the attitudes and habits that affected their well-being. This goal encompassed the need to detect and relieve symptoms but also transcended it by its concern for health. However, neither physicians nor patients embraced this ideal.

Physicians focused on finding diseases in places within the body, and to this end they enthusiastically and skillfully applied a growing twentieth-century technology. Treating illness was their job and the mission filled their day, a viewpoint confirmed by the well-known Boston physician Maurice Fremont-Smith in a mid-1950s comment on the typical response of physicians to patients seeking a periodic checkup: "The doctor is apt to say he has no time for this type of health survey." He had acquired this attitude in the 1920s during his training at Massachusetts General Hospital: "What I wanted then were sick people who would get well and be grateful, or cases of advanced disease with good abnormal physical signs for differential diagnosis and teaching purposes. Many physicians still feel the same way about patients with little or nothing apparently the matter with them."[19]

The public's view of the physician's role reinforced this position. You went to the doctor when you felt sick. Feeling well was a prescription for staying away. The additional factor of saving money as a reason for rationing doctor visits did not necessarily weigh heavily in the decision to forgo periodic examinations. For example, when the Metropolitan Life Insurance Company offered them to policyholders over an eight-year period (1914 to 1921) at no cost, only 2.5 percent of those eligible for the benefit used it.[20] To most people, being healthy meant cultivating sound habits of living. And the knowledge, interest, and responsibility to oversee this goal seemed to reside outside of medicine's orbit as concerns of individuals and families, assisted by cultural and religious mores and plain common sense.

But those persuaded by the arguments of the periodic examination movement to seek out physicians to keep them well often were disappointed by the encounter, as illustrated by the account of a patient in the mid-1950s: "In the last three years, I have gone to two different doctors for *complete* physicals. Neither one of them made any motion to go beyond taking my blood pressure and giving an ear to my heart and lungs.... Maybe if clinics were set up for checkups for people who think they are in good health, doctors wouldn't be so annoyed at having their precious time taken up by unbroken bones and healthy tissues."[21]

In the 1950s an alternative to fulfilling the promise of the periodic examination by physicians appeared that had limited but more achievable goals – mass population screening for several diseases at a time conducted by public health departments. Screening entails testing people for disorders they are at risk of getting and identifying them at an early stage of development, when they have not yet generated symptoms. The accuracy of the screening test depends on its ability to detect a high proportion of those who have the targeted disorder (low false-negative rate), but without excessively attributing the disease to those who are well (low false-positive rate). There also should be evidence that early-detection programs produce clear benefits, such as gaining better outcomes in people found to harbor a disease in its early stages than patients in whom the disorder is discovered later through general medical care.[22]

As with the periodic examination, the idea behind screening is to actively encourage the public to seek out the service when feeling well; unlike it, screening is a limited technological intervention, which requires a follow-up of positive results consisting of further testing and examination by doctors to get a definitive diagnosis. Thus, screening for a disease is distinguishable from its diagnosis by the level of certitude attached to the result. While the same technology can be employed both for screening and for diagnosis, the purpose of its use and the context within which it is applied can give the same agent a different value.

During the first half of the twentieth century, campaigns were waged to convince the public to be screened with a particular technology for a particular disease. A prime example of this is the X-ray, which became not only the premier diagnostic technology of that time but also its most visible agent of screening. In the 1940s and 1950s, mobile vans that housed X-ray machines and were sponsored by public health agencies crisscrossed America. The vans parked in neighborhoods for several days and screened people without cost for chest diseases, most notably tuberculosis. Later, physicians read the X-rays and mailed a report of the findings to its subject, with advice for getting follow-up care if needed. Syphilis was another major disease for which a blood test, the Wasserman test, was developed in 1906 and used widely in the United States by public health departments both as a mandatory screening procedure of couples before marriage and as a means to locate the illness in vulnerable segments of the population such as pregnant women. The campaigns to alert and inform the public about the dangers of such disorders used posters having strong graphic imagery and slogans to emphasize their messages. They became an increasingly important aspect of public health preventive efforts (Figures 15 and 16).

However, in the 1950s single campaigns directed at a single disease were challenged by a new concept, multiphasic population screening, whose popularity grew as the decade wore on. It bundled tests together in a technological recreation of the periodic examination but without the need for a doctor visit. Adopting the strategy of the mobile X-ray unit, these tests were brought to the people. Screening booths were set up at neighborhood and county fairs, in local schools and in health departments, places where people went for enjoyment or were nearby and convenient to reach. These bundled screening tests also consumed less time and expense than did periodic examinations.

The tests themselves were directed at detecting major ailments such as heart disease, diabetes, and cancer, for which new screening techniques had been developed in the 1940s. Multiple testing had the additional virtue of eliminating the anxieties generated by screening campaigns directed at a single illness. Such campaigns often focused on the dire consequences of the illness and the failure to get tested, and thus ironically generated fear about disorder in the public they were intended to influence and thereby subverted the success of their message.

Early studies found multiphasic screening effective, such as one in 1951 that uncovered significant disorders in more than half of those tested, among which were diabetes, syphilis, tuberculosis, cancer, high

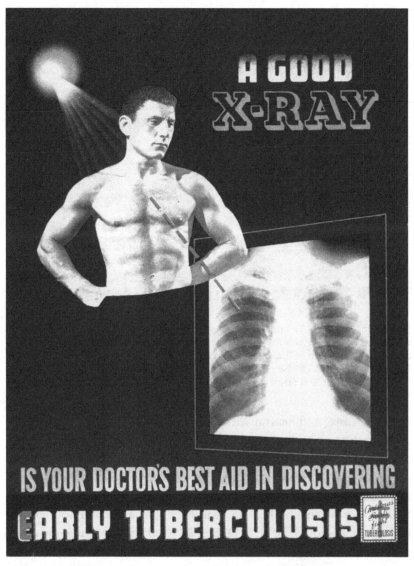

Figure 15. A poster urging preventive chest X-rays (ca. 1940). The illustration depicts the power of X-rays to pierce the body's outer structure and accurately reveal its inner condition, emphasizes the vulnerability to tuberculosis of even a young and muscular person who may harbor it unknowingly, and thereby seeks to spur preventive action by the public who views it. Reprinted with permission © 2008 American Lung Association. For more information about the American Lung Association or to support the work it does, call 1-800-LUNG-USA (1-800-586-4872) or log on to www.lungusa.org.

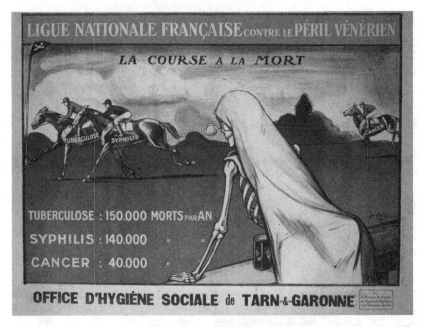

Figure 16. *La course à la mort* (The race with death). From the rail of a track, Death watches a race of three prevalent diseases, in an illustration informing the public of their danger and annual toll of life, in a readily-grasped and vivid manner. Drawn by Charles Emmanuel Jockelet, Ligue Nationale Française contre le Péril Vénérien, France, ca. 1926. Courtesy of the National Library of Medicine.

blood pressure, and heart disease.[23] But after a decade, use of the concept began to wane because screening programs were not dependably connected to follow-up diagnosis and therapy. And even though the screening tests generally were free, the follow-up care was not. A 1967 comment by a Georgia Department of Health official illustrates the follow-up problem: "When we went back into a community that we had screened a couple of years before, we would find the same old cases of T.B., less the ones that had died, plus new ones. To me, screening is no objective in itself, and just finding cases and dropping them has no value."[24]

However, screening did not go away. Throughout the rest of the twentieth century an exponential growth of new screening tests and efforts to apply them occurred, reflecting technological developments and the increasing assumption that early detection of disease is beneficial.[25] Among the major screening efforts were ones to detect cancers, disease-causing genetic abnormalities, heart and blood-vessel disorders, and chronic diseases such as osteoporosis, as well as to assess health and disabilities in children and elderly people. Such preventive testing increasingly was used in the work of physicians and managed-care organizations, thus integrating its ordering and interpreting. But this growth produced a host of medical, social, and ethical issues, which increased debate and uncertainty about screening. How to weigh the dangers and advantages of aggressively treating a person identified through a screening program to have a nonprogressive or slowly developing lesion, which might remain localized and never develop into a full-blown disease? In such circumstances, is the morbidity and mortality connected with the therapy worse or better for the individual or population affected by the disease? And should society mount screening programs for people with these kinds of lesions in the first place? Such dilemmas demonstrate the need to fully understand the natural history of the disorder for which a screening program is proposed before it is publicly implemented.[26]

And what to do as genetic testing identifies individuals who carry mutations that may raise their risk of contracting a serious disease such as breast or ovarian cancer, or can accurately foretell that an individual will contract a dread disorder in the distant future, such as the neurologically disabling and life-threatening Huntington's disease? In the first instance, should individuals choose a life of repeated genetic screenings to catch the disorder in an early phase, or have their breasts or ovaries removed surgically to prevent its appearance totally? As for the second example, deciding whether to learn that you have Huntington's disease years before it will appear is a life-changing decision as profound as medical choices can get.

False-positive results also received greater attention. Again, these were circumstances in which one screening test declared the presence of a disease only to have a repeated evaluation with the same or a different test reverse the verdict. Which result to believe? And how best to help individuals cope with the contradictory findings? Too often, busy physicians giving out the good news that a repeat test is normal do not explore adequately the fears and feelings of the individual who, most likely, will be asked to have the test again in the following year and possibly relive the earlier experience. Such issues do not discredit the use of screening but demonstrate the perplexing questions it raises, the novel situations it creates, and the complicated counseling it requires.

The success of twentieth-century screening to locate diseases in their bodily lairs when they have barely begun their existence and knock them out with powerful technological remedies has been among the factors keeping medicine from having a strong concern with the determinants of health. The structuralist theory of disease, which has oriented and anchored medical thinking from the nineteenth century and into the present, essentially depicts health as the absence of disease. Is it not a common experience when examined by doctors today to be assured one is healthy if signs of illness are absent?

The limits of this generic medical viewpoint began to emerge in the 1940s as new autopsy studies cast doubt on the concept of normality as freedom from anatomical defects. They revealed lesions in people who had never experienced symptoms or illness from them and suggested the need for a different vision of illness, particularly as it concerned the issue of work. Studies conducted by industry at this time revealed that physically handicapped workers were as productive as and took no more time off for sickness or personal reasons than their nonhandicapped colleagues, and indeed could surpass them in productivity. To account for this outcome, some theorized that a disability can become a stimulus to overcompensation of the personality. Taking such factors into account, a 1940 article in the *Journal of the American Medical Association* defined physical fitness in the widest sense to mean "the ability to perform productive and continuous work."[27]

The notion that a state of health is compatible with significant structural bodily damage remains outside of mainstream medical thinking. But it is crucial to replace the prevailing concept of health with one that more readily speaks to who people are and how they live. Although it was wrong in its biological explanations, the environmentalist concept embodied by the humoral theory grasped the reality of health and illness in a way that the structuralist concept that followed it did not. The environmentalist concept explains the states of health and illness in a single unifying concept – adaptability. How in this theory does one get sick? Through an inability to adapt to one or more of the natural, biological, or social environments in which the person lives. Adaptive failure, in turn, creates an instability in the functioning of the body and the person, which is experienced as illness. Recovery to wellness occurs when the ability to sustain a relationship of stability with one's encircling environments returns. This can happen even if the body continues to be damaged and threatened, as in the case of disabilities produced by war, by chronic disease such as arthritis, or by life-threatening disease such as cancer or AIDS. Health in the face of disease is possible and widely demonstrated by those whose productive and fulfilling life continues in its presence, but is not a concept that fits the anatomic and structuralist-based thinking of medicine. This state of being thus requires a vision that accommodates its realities. And it is to this matter that we now turn.

Over the centuries in which humoral theory reigned, the powerful connection it made between illness and health was undermined by the fallacies of its biological explanation of these states, which the structuralist concept challenged and got right, at least in part. Illness is often a product of structural damage and the changes in function that causes, which produce the feelings and disabilities experienced as symptoms. And research has demonstrated a host of agents, from bacteria to industrial toxins, that can create bodily damage.

But it is at the nineteenth-century junction when structuralism took over from environmentalism that a crucial separation occurred – medicine began increasingly to bifurcate into two basic branches. One branch focused on the care of individual patients using the powerful diagnostic and therapeutic tools that the structuralist concept inspired. The other, while applying structuralist concepts and therapies in its work, maintained a steadfast focus on environments as the basic soils within which disease-causing or health-producing stimuli and agents could flourish, and made its concern the populations of people who lived within them. In the nineteenth century, this branch formally organized and professionalized a discipline separate from medicine that came to be called public health. It concerned itself with long-standing environmental interests such as water quality, sanitation, preventive therapies applied to populations such as disease immunization, the effects of living conditions and nutrition on health and illness, and so forth. These actions now were undertaken increasingly by health officials, formally appointed and paid by municipal and state governments to oversee and enforce health regulations, like John Pintard, the first American to hold such a post when he was made city inspector of health in New York in 1804. As their numbers grew, health officers and others concerned with community health sponsored national conventions to discuss pressing issues, activities that were the formative basis of the American Public Health Association, established in 1872.[28]

In the twentieth century, public health added a discipline that elaborated an innovative vision for creating and sustaining health and aptly called *health promotion*. Health had always been a concern of public health, but this discipline took its study to a higher level. An important influence on its development was evidence from the branch of public health that examines causal agents of health and illness in populations, epidemiology, which demonstrated new linkages between health and factors in the social environment. Another was the World Health Organization (WHO), created as a branch of the United Nations. In 1948 the WHO issued an enlarged definition of health as "physical, mental and social well-being, not merely the absence of disease and infirmity,"[29] and subsequently sponsored international meetings having health-related agendas. However, recognition of health promotion as a distinct field came from a 1974 monograph issued by the Canadian minister of health and welfare, Mark Lalonde: *A New Perspective on the Health of Canadians*. Its message was enlarged in the 1986 Ottawa Charter for Health Promotion, sponsored by the WHO and promulgated at the field's first international conference. The charter enumerated fundamental determinants of health like adequate food and income, as well as strategies both to strengthen environments supporting health and to provide people with skills to preserve their health. It described health promotion as "the process of enabling people to increase control over, and to improve their health," and described health as "a resource for everyday life...a positive concept emphasizing social and personal resources as well as physical capabilities," a view elaborated on by public health scholar Lester Breslow. He proposed delineating and measuring specific capacities to strengthen this resource and thus the ability of individuals to maintain a stable relationship with the environments around them. For example, tests of physiological function such as performance on an exercise treadmill, or of biochemical status such as cholesterol levels could be used to measure not only one's potential for becoming sick but also for achieving health. Similar evaluations could be made in the social sphere of life such as the strength of a person's social network, and in the mental domain such as the ability to maintain a positive mood and a good working memory. The evaluations were steps to interventions that improved these capacities which, he declared "exemplify the kind of reserves needed not only to maintain balance in life's exigencies but also to exercise the potential for enjoyment . . . whether one's interests be reading, climbing mountains, hearing music, [or] spending time with family.[30]

In the year of the charter's publication, the WHO advanced the idea of promoting health in defined settings that focused its goals and actions, as the organization began its internationally successful program Healthy Cities. And as the twentieth century ended, public health scholars and practitioners were emphasizing the importance to health of settings like schools, hospitals, and workplaces. This focus gave health promotion a broadly ecological perspective and redirected its gaze, as noted in a recent work, "from individual, behavioral risk factors to the more distal determinants of health beyond their personal control. Organizational settings provide a middle ground between individual behavior (the primary focus of past efforts) and higher levels of social organization beyond the grasp of practitioners, as a place to come to grips with the determinants of health. The ecological perspective presents health as a product of the interdependence between the individual and subsystems of the ecosystem . . . [which] may include family, peer groups, organizations, community, culture, and physical and social environment."[31] Accordingly, health promotion follows the ancient Greek interest in how the relation of people with the environments within which they live influence their health. But it goes further in stressing the need for society to both empower and assist individuals and communities to attain health.

Synthesizing these strands of historical thinking, health emerges as the inherent, self-nourished, socially and medically-influenced endowment of individuals to adaptively meet the challenges and opportunities presented to them by the multiple environments that encompass their lives.

In the late twentieth century, as the environmentalist-centered field of health promotion grew within the hospitable framework of public health, so did the structuralist view of health and illness continue to flourish in medicine. It was shaped by extraordinary developments in genetic science, which culminated in a 2001 publication of the sequence of the 3 billion base pairs that compose the human genome – a line of research referred to as "mapping the genome." However, this map did not reveal how the base pairs varied among people or the correlation between particular segments of the genome and different diseases or human traits. Recent research has helped fill these lacunae, such as with what are called haplotype maps. They identify about a half million segments of DNA called haplotype bins, which function as zip codes to locate changes in genetic structure that affect human traits and illness.

With such tools, the pace of discovering genetic indices associated with significant common ailments has become so swift that a group of genetic scientists labeled it "the Genomics Gold Rush." Just weeks before their 2007 article bearing this title appeared, its authors noted the publication of a bundle of studies that revealed genetic markers linked with human susceptibility to "the most common diseases, ranging from acute lymphoblastic leukemia, the most important pediatric cancer, to obesity, type 2 diabetes mellitus, and coronary heart disease, which collectively affect nearly a billion individuals worldwide. The breakneck pace of discovery will be continuing in the months ahead, with anticipated findings for many cancers, cardiovascular diseases, and neurological diseases. In aggregate, these studies have the potential to radically change medicine."[32]

But this work has conceptual and practical limitations. These scientists wrote: "Like the initial map of the genome in 2001, the biomedical research community is still much too 'anatomic'centric, given the recent ability to identify DNA markers associated with important human diseases, but little knowledge that relates these DNA variants with the specific, molecular pathways that induce susceptibility. Current gaps in explaining the genomic basis of disease may ultimately reflect that complexity outside of common . . . [base-pair variants] is important."[33] The vocabulary employed to describe and discuss genes, using concepts like maps and bins that direct us to the location of things in places, reveals the influence of structuralist thinking in genetics. However, the authors of "The Genomics Gold Rush" article suggest, exploring the complex environments with which genes interact is needed to explain their role in disease. Thus, the focus of anatomic study has shifted over the past three centuries to increasingly smaller units of analysis – from the organ to the cell to the gene – but this work has continued to center medicine on the same fundamental question: *Ubi est morbus?* or, Where is the disease?

These developments make it essential for medicine and public health to place health and illness within a conceptual framework, in which understanding the conditions creating health for individuals and populations receive coequal study and status with those producing illness, and in which a broadened array of factors explaining and producing these basic states of being undergird analysis and practice in the health professions. The best approach to accomplish this, and to integrate structuralist thinking and actions into a broader framework, is the environmental-adaptive concept of disease and wellness. However, an important ingredient in creating a theoretical concordance on the nature of health and illness is a political concordance between medicine and public health.

The prospects for cooperation between the two professions have recently improved in the United States, where they have begun to heal rifts that widened during the twentieth century in the aftermath of their earlier intellectual and work-related parting. In this period, the two professions not only established separate schools and spheres of work but also were antagonistic when one trespassed too closely on the other's bailiwick. In the 1950s, for example, physicians bristled over the screening of patients by public health departments and accused them of encroaching on their terrain of practice.[34]

By the 1990s the divisive politics between them and the damage to the health-care system had become serious enough for their leaders to forge a cooperative relationship through a movement they inaugurated in 1994 called the Medicine/Public Health Initiative. Early in that year, the initiative's steering committee met in the nation's capital to forge its agenda. It was hosted by the American Medical Association (AMA) but chaired by Eugene Feingold, the American Public Health Association (APHA) president – an arrangement meant to symbolize their new relationship. I was there when Feingold opened the session. Reacting with great feeling to the significance of the event, he said, and I can only paraphrase his comment: "I never would have dreamed that a president of the APHA would ever stand in the Washington headquarters of the

American Medical Association to preside at a meeting between them."
All present recognized the moment's deep meaning.

Two years after its founding, the initiative held a first-of-its-kind
convocation in Chicago of some four hundred state and national leaders
of medicine and public health to galvanize cooperative actions to benefit
the country. Chaired by the leadership of the AMA and APHA, the
conference was addressed by dignitaries such as C. Everett Koop, the
former U.S. surgeon general, and the U.S. secretary of health and human
services, Donna Shalala. In her remarks, the secretary likened public
health and medicine "to trains on parallel tracks with windows facing
in opposite directions looking out at different terrain." She praised their
intended collaboration and declared the success of their efforts was
crucial in securing the nation's well-being.[35] After the meeting work
to realize this collaborative spirit through research, educational, and
health-care service projects occurred all over the country.

The initiative had a strong and effective influence until the start of
the twenty-first century, in which it has had a much lower profile and
level of activity, but it has continued to encourage cooperation between
public health and medicine in the states. While it did not achieve the
concordance of the two professions for which its founders had hoped,
the initiative healed old wounds and committed them to collaborative
efforts.

A significant opportunity to demonstrate the possibilities of this part-
nership is forging a conceptual framework that not only links health
and illness, but reintroduces into the relationship between doctor and
patient a robust focus on health based on comprehensively exploring
its biological and social characteristics and determinants, objective and
subjective measures, clinical dimensions, and so forth.[36] Anchored by
medicine and public health, the views and experience of other health
professions and consumers should be brought to this effort. A unified
theory based on an environmental/adaptive perspective that rebalances
the attention health and illness receive in the care of patients and populations has the potential of substantially bettering their lives. For this
approach connects the efforts of public health practitioners working
to improve the natural and social conditions of human existence, with

the activities of medical practitioners seeking to heal and sustain the biological and psychological functions of individuals. It provides a foundation for the evolution of a health care system that comprehensively addresses essential individual and social vulnerabilities and needs, and whose lowered technological emphasis enhances its cost-reducing potential.

8

THE TECHNOLOGICAL
TRANSFORMATION OF BIRTH

The eighteenth-century obstetrician William Smellie confronted a dilemma. Women feared the forceps, a technology newly revealed to the medical world, with which babies unable to exit the womb in a natural way could be safely grasped by the head and delivered. The dilemma was finding a way to apply them in cases needing their help. In his 1752 treatise on birth, Smellie published a solution. He instructed the doctor to hide the blades in his side pockets during prebirth activities. When the time to deliver the baby arrived, Smellie wrote,

Let him spread the sheet that hangs over the bed, upon his lap, and under the cover, take out and dispose the blades on each side of the patient; by which means he will often be able to deliver with the forceps, without their being perceived by the woman herself, or any other of the assistants. Some people pin a sheet to each shoulder, and throw the other end over the bed, that they may be the more effectually concealed from the view of those who are present: but this method is apt to confine and embarrass the operator. At any rate, as women are commonly frightened at the very name of an instrument, it is advisable to conceal them as much as possible.[1]

Childbirth, a transcendent personal and social event, has generated conflict throughout history about the values, rites, and procedures that should bound it. In the past four centuries a central feature of this conflict has been disagreement about the advantages and dangers conferred by technology on birth. Technology changed not only the physical experience of birth but also the decision-making power of those involved in it, and thereby it profoundly affected the event. This chapter explores these developments.

As the seventeenth century began, routine childbirth was not associated with medical technology. It was based in the home, to which women, having both personal and clinical experience with birth as well as relationships with the birthing woman, came to provide care and comfort. Childbirth and rearing were central features of life for a woman of this time, who in an ordinary span of life bore an average of seven children. As Levitt noted: "Women suffered through agonies and dangers of birth together, sought each others' support, and shared the relief of successful deliveries and the grief of unsuccessful ones. This 'social childbirth' experience united women."[2]

In this group, the woman with the widest clinical experience was the midwife, a figure associated with childbirth from biblical times. Her views generally dominated the scene, and her clinical style at its best was cautious: to observe much, to intervene little, to encourage as needed, to wait, and to be there. In the mid-fifteenth century, the German municipality of Regensburg had initiated the regulation of midwives in Europe, evaluating their character and skills and forbidding actions such as performing abortions and magical rites. By the seventeenth century in England, formal training for a novice could mean up to seven years of apprenticeship to an experienced midwife before she could display the symbol of the calling, a cradle. These professed midwives stood at the top of their field and practiced mainly in urban settings, where earnings would likely reflect their training. Most rewarding was treating royalty, as the leading French midwife Madame Peronne demonstrated. She received a one-hundred-pound living allowance and a three-hundred-pound birthing fee in 1630 for attending Henrietta Maria, wife of Charles I.[3]

But generally the lives of midwives were hard; their incomes were low; and for some, their work was largely altruistic. In rural eighteenth-century France, for example, midwives were seldom paid and then mainly with food. They traveled long distances in all kinds of weather and at any time of day. They were granted authority by the church to give emergency baptism if fetal death seemed imminent. The learning of these rural midwives was often transmitted in families rather than gained through formal education. Books for midwives that provided brief and simple accounts of the birth process, written by physicians and surgeons, had begun to appear in the seventeenth century. They were of little help to rural midwives, for many could not read. But from handed-down and personal experience they closely observed labor, following the fetus's position in the uterus, helping the mother find comfortable positions, maintaining pleasant room temperature, providing sustenance to the woman, and using herbs to hasten delivery. However, in situations of a stalled birth at times the midwife engaged in actions that were dangerous. They could push on the abdomen and cause fetal or maternal harm, or pull on the head or presenting limb of the fetus and create hemorrhage. And after birth, they could risk injuring the mother by pulling out the placenta from impatience at its slow natural delivery.[4]

Thus, while helpful with normal labor by virtue of a watching and waiting presence and attitude, when this approach failed, particularly in the face of impending crises that delayed birth and threatened fetal and maternal life, practitioners with different learning and experience were needed. And this experience most likely was possessed by the surgeon. As noted in earlier chapters, surgery was split from medicine when medical education was located in the scholastic and bookish environment of emerging medieval universities, and surgical training was acquired mainly through apprenticeship. Surgeons' manual skills and knowledge of anatomy and instruments gave surgeons practical learning to intervene in situations when the natural contractions of labor and the efforts of the midwife were unavailing, and passage of the fetus from the womb was obstructed.

Obstructed labor could be caused by a narrow pelvis or a large baby, both of which impeded the transit of the fetus through the birth canal; or by malpositioning of the infant in the uterus, in which the infant's largest and most solid part, the head, was not positioned to lead the way out of the womb (Figure 17). In the face of such conditions the different learning and experience of the surgeon provided the hope of avoiding tragedy. To facilitate live delivery, in cases where a malpositioned baby either lay crosswise within the uterus or where the feet or buttocks were leading its exit from the womb (defined as a breech presentation), the surgeons could attempt the procedure of version, a repositioning of the baby in the uterus. They did this manually and/or resorted to instruments such as the fillet (used to place a band around the body or a limb) or the more dangerous blunt hook. These were used to draw the baby down and through the birth canal, a difficult process with uncertain outcomes. But the infant tragically and hopelessly stuck in

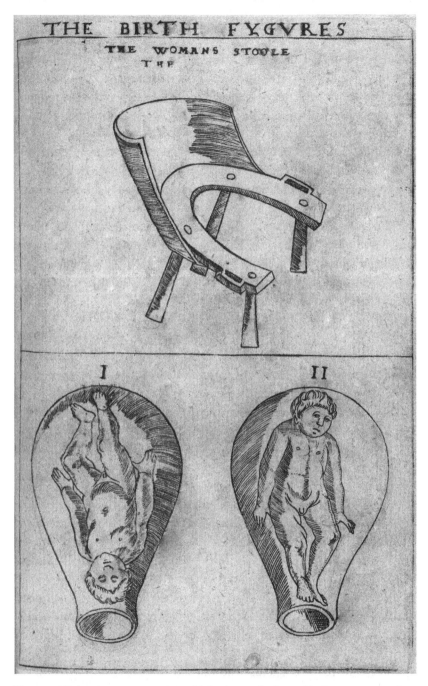

Figure 17. Before contemporary times, birth often took place with the woman seated on specially designed chairs or stools such as shown in the illustration at the top. Beneath the stool on the left is a baby positioned in the normal headfirst or vertex position, and on the right is one in a problematic feetfirst or breech position. From Thomas Raynald, *The Byrth of Mankynde*, 1545. Courtesy of Wellcome Library, London.

the uterus was instrumentally sectioned by the surgeon in an extreme effort to save the life of the mother; or the desperate act of opening the uterus of a mother – the operation of cesarean section – attempted to save the baby if the mother had died or to save the mother if the baby had. It was rarely tried or successful.

Yet access to the hope the surgeon might provide carried a double price for the woman in labor – she faced not only the danger of aggressive therapeutic manipulation applied to herself and her fetus but also the despair of having members of a male-dominated profession invade the privacy of her body, which the collegium of female attendants maintained and protected. Laget wrote: "the fear of being indecent, the fear of being dishonored, the fear of being seen in the throes of suffering – these great ageless concerns were at the core of the debate over 'the indecency of having men deliver women.'"[5]

The invention of the obstetric forceps led to a series of developments that changed the relationship, settings, and experiences of the birth process. It did so by permitting a medical attendant to replace the natural powers of the body to accomplish this most personally significant and publicly visible aspect of pregnancy – expelling a baby into the world. By increasing distrust in natural bodily forces to bring the baby from the womb and substituting a power given to the birth attendant by technology – beginning with the obstetric forceps – the physical, social, and psychological context of delivering children was transformed. The obstetric forceps opened the way to accepting other technological advances intended to improve the chances for a well mother and baby to emerge from a pregnancy. But the price of the benefits was a gradual transfer of authority over birthing from the mother and female friends and midwife attending her to a male-centered medical collegium, which created a vision of birth as a medical rather than a natural condition and sociocultural event, and gradually changed the site of care from the home to the hospital.

Forceps to remove a fetus who did not survive in the womb have existed since ancient times. But one constructed to accomplish the more delicate task of extracting a living baby did not appear until 1554, when Jacob Rueff published a work that described and illustrated such an instrument. The rationale for the innovation was finding a more effective and safer alternative to the hands to deliver a baby by grasping its head. However, there is no evidence that Rueff's forceps were applied in practice, most likely because the design was inadequate for the purpose. The two blades were fixed together, like a pliers, compelling the user to place them on the sides of the head simultaneously, a difficult maneuver. Further, the curve of the blades was inadequate to embrace the head firmly and provide the traction needed for delivery.

A forceps without these failings appeared in the following century. It featured two appropriately curved and unjoined blades that could be applied to the head individually, and then secured together to extract the infant. The forceps were developed by a member of an English medical family of surgeons and physicians practicing obstetrics, the Chamberlens, who shrouded their use in secrecy and passed them among themselves from generation to generation for more than a century. The family's life in England began with William Chamberlen, a French Huguenot who immigrated there in 1569. He named two of his sons Peter, Peter the Elder and Peter the Younger. The most likely inventor of the forceps was the Elder (circa 1560–1631). He was surgeon to the wife of James I, Queen Anne, and attended births in the royal family. Peter the Younger (circa 1572–1620) also practiced surgery and midwifery. His son, a third Peter Chamberlen, known as Dr. Peter (1601–1683), became a physician who also delivered children using the forceps. He in turn, passed the invention on to his sons, three of whom were physicians.[6]

One of them, Hugh (1630–1726), confirmed that the Chamberlens indeed had a unique way of treating difficult births but did not disclose its nature. The revelation appeared in a 1673 translation he made of François Mauriceau's treatise on diseases of pregnancy, which Chamberlen titled *The Accomplish't Midwife* and that proved influential for midwifery education in England. He writes in the preface:

In the 17th Chapter of the second Book, my Author [Mauriceau] justifies the fastning Hooks in the Head of a Child that comes right, and yet because of some Difficulty or Disproportion cannot pass; which I confess has been, and is yet the Practice of the most expert Artists in Midwifery, not only in England, but throughout Europe; and has much caused the Report, that where a Man comes [to deliver a child], one or both must necessarily die; and is the reason of forbearing to send, till the Child is dead, or the Mother dying. But

I can neither approve of that Practice, nor those Delays; because my Father, Brothers, and my Self (tho none else in Europe as I know) have, by God's Blessing and our Industry, attained to, and long practised a way to deliver Women in this Case, without any Prejudice to them or their Infants; tho all others (being obliged, for want of such an Expedient, to use the Common way) do, and must endanger, if not destroy one or both with Hooks.[7]

Declaring the promise of his family's innovation to humanity was that "a labor may be dispatched (on the least difficulty) with fewer pains and sooner, to the great advantage and without danger both of woman and child," Hugh then defends the Chamberlens' decision to keep knowledge of it to themselves: "I will now take leave to offer an apology for not publishing the secret I mention we have to extract children without hooks, where other artists use them, viz., there being my Father and two Brothers living, that practise this art, I cannot esteem it my own to dispose of nor publish it without injury to them; and think I have not been unservicable to my country, altho I do but inform them that the forementioned three persons of our family and myself, can serve in these extremities, with greater safety than others."[8]

But how to explain the Chamberlens' success in maintaining a family secret through much of the seventeenth and up to the early eighteenth century? It was customary when male surgeons participated in childbirth to do so under the cover of a sheet tied around the neck, to maintain some degree of privacy and prevent the surgical intervention from alarming the birthing woman (Figure 18). This practice may explain in part how forceps use could be concealed by the Chamberlens, as Smellie's comments on the practice that introduced this chapter show. But there are allegations in the literature that the Chamberlens went further by sequestering the forceps in a box carried into the birthing room, blindfolding the woman in labor, excluding everyone else from the room before opening the box, and bringing family and other attendants back only after delivering the baby. However, what really happened remains unclear.

There also is considerable speculation about how the Chamberlen forceps were revealed to the world but no definitive evidence. Hugh apparently tried to sell the secret, but it is uncertain whether he succeeded. In the first half of the eighteenth century, a variety of obstetric forceps having forms somewhat different from that of the Chamberlens' had emerged in Belgium, France, and England, but the question remains,

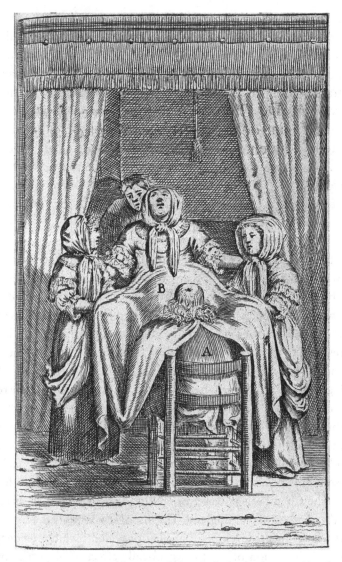

Figure 18. A male practitioner delivering a baby wholly by touch, to avoid embarrassing the woman or alarming her should the need for using instruments arise. From S. Janson. *Korte en Bonding verhandeling, van de voortteelingen 't Kinderbaren.* Amsterdam, 1711. Courtesy of Wellcome Library, London.

How did precise knowledge about them spread? Some things we know. The community of midwives and medical men were aware the Chamberlens used some form of technology. Midwives in particular were well acquainted with the Chamberlens' practices, because they called for their help in difficult births. Thus, replying to a proposal by Dr. Peter in 1633 to organize and educate them, the midwives responded: "Dr. Chamberlen's work and the work belonging to midwives are contrary one to the other for he delivers none without the use of instruments by extraordinary violence in desperate occasions, which women never practised nor desyred for they have neither parts nor hands for that art."[9] The remark not only confirms an awareness of the Chamberlens' use of technology but also reflects the custom in midwifery practice to shun the use of instruments. A year later, a letter to Dr. Peter by the College of Physicians condemned his proposal too, and took note of his "use of iron instruments," another sign that rumors existed about the Chamberlens' innovation.[10]

Most likely, then, cumulative factors were at play in gradually providing the medical world with specific information about the forceps: from women on whom the forceps were applied and family members at the birth site who might have gotten wind of what was used; from surgeons, physicians, and midwives who had medical contact with the Chamberlens; from the Chamberlens themselves through unwitting disclosures; and from individuals to whom they might have sold the secret and who in turn revealed it to others. Such leaked evidence, allied to a growing interest in childbirth by physicians and surgeons, and the resulting accumulation of anatomical and physiological knowledge about it, probably produced the phenomenon of simultaneous discovery, when an idea spreads in society and leads a number of individuals toward a particular finding or invention within the same period.[11] A conclusion to these events occurred in the early nineteenth century when forceps used by the Chamberlens were found hidden beneath floorboards in a house they had owned in England. The discovery not only demonstrated how the instrument developed but also provided tangible evidence of the family's invention of the therapeutically effective obstetric forceps (Figure 19).

An ethical question remains: what justified the Chamberlens to keep knowledge of an instrument with the lifesaving potential of the obstetric forceps from the community of practitioners concerned with birth for more than a century? A viewpoint about invention and discovery foreign to modern concepts of disclosure prevailed in the seventeenth century. Knowledge was widely viewed as pivotal to understand and control nature and, as Wilbanks puts it, "If one earned a sizeable amount, one

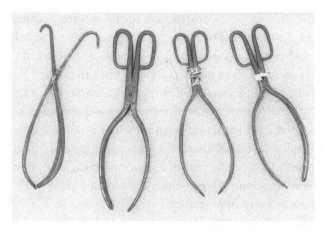

Figure 19. Four pairs of Chamberlen forceps discovered in 1813 beneath an attic trapdoor in Woodham Mortimer Hall, the English home of the third Peter Chamberlen (Dr. Peter) that was sold by the family in 1715. They illustrate the evolution of the instrument's design. All the instruments are appropriately curved to embrace the baby's head, but, except for the first model, their blades are well-separated, thus reducing the possibility of putting undue pressure on it. A key to their successful use was developing a dependable means of locking the blades together to have adequate traction to extract the baby. Viewing the forceps from left to right, in the first and flawed design, the blades are riveted together, making their introduction into the birth canal difficult. The remaining designs have separate blades, with increasingly better means of aligning and fastening them once the practitioner was ready to draw out the baby. Thus, the second design had a pivot on one blade and a hole in the other, but aligning and locking them in place was difficult. The third and fourth designs used tape passed through holes, and this simple remedy proved the easiest and most effective way to secure them together. From *The Chamberlen Forceps*, London, Royal College of Obstetricians and Gynecologists Press, 2003. © Royal College of Obstetricians and Gynaecologists, reproduced with permission.

had a nest egg to be carefully guarded."[12] This view allowed medical innovators to remain silent about their treatments in order to earn profits. Testimony of satisfied patients rather than externally validated confirmation of a remedy's effects was the norm. An example is what were known in eighteenth-century France as *remèdes secrets*. These were therapies exploited commercially by their innovators, both physicians and nonmedical healers. Remedies that were drugs, for example, were not registered in the pharmacopoeia kept by apothecaries. They were so prevalent that the French government tried to regulate them. By the end of the eighteenth century, while medical opinion in France against such secrecy was rising, some physicians continued to defend the right of an inventor to exploit a discovery for monetary gain by concealing its nature from clinicians and other commercial rivals. It was a matter of property rights trumping social needs.[13]

Once the idea for and construction of the forceps became publicly available in the first third of the eighteenth century, it was taken up by surgeons and physicians interested in childbirth, and during this century the number and types of this technology proliferated.[14] Some of the most ardent advocates urged a cautious and judicious use of the forceps, recognizing their ability to produce great good but also their great destructive potential to the fetus and woman in labor. One of them, William Smellie, declared that "the forceps in general should not be used, especially in the early part of a man's practice, except only on the most urgent occasions."[15] But others could not resist their use and applied them at every opportunity.

A question remains about the role played by forceps in replacing female birth attendants with male practitioners from surgery and medicine. Women were ambivalent about having the "jaws of iron," as many called the forceps, placed in their body. For doing so could be painful, injurious, and carried disturbing associations with dreaded surgical interventions. Yet they also were drawn to the aid the forceps offered in making labor shorter and less dangerous for themselves and their baby.

Given their ambivalence, more than forceps were needed for expectant mothers to choose a new class of attendants to deliver their children. And that *more* was a growing belief in the general capability of medicine and surgery, which began to develop in the eighteenth century. As Loudon wrote: "It was the public, the women themselves, who in substantial numbers deliberately chose to engage a medical practitioner when there were plenty of skilled and capable midwives of high reputation to choose from Their choice must have had something to do with the rise in the status of the medical practitioner." Part of this rise was catalyzed by substantive advances in understanding pregnancy and labor, such as the anatomical changes of the uterus during pregnancy; the character of normal labor; dividing the process of labor into three stages; and improving the management of its crucial third stage through accurate knowledge of how the placenta normally separated from the uterus. Such advances spurred eighteenth-century physicians and surgeons to view birth as a logical extension of their ordinary sphere of care. They found, too, that delivering children gained them community trust and expanded their practice. However, until the late nineteenth century, medical and surgical associations resisted making childbirth an acceptable feature of professional life. In England in the earlier part of the century, for example, the College of Physicians believed it was ungentlemanly for a doctor to deliver babies, and the College of Surgeons wished its members to focus on basic surgery and not be involved with birth.[16]

In summary, in the eighteenth century, the collegium of female birth attendants whose knowledge derived largely from personal experience and apprenticeship learning was joined increasingly by male practitioners. They had limited practical familiarity with birth but possessed technologies and anatomical learning that gave them a therapeutic edge in meeting its more dangerous problems, which might daunt the midwife. And their professional standing seemed to confer an advantage over the midwife – even though they lacked her experience and gender identity (Figure 20).

Accepting childbirth as an aspect of medicine during the nineteenth century was advanced by other innovations. The most critical were means to reduce the pain of labor and prevent dangerous diseases that could accompany birth, most notably puerperal fever. The use of anesthetics came first. A significant barrier to their introduction was incredulity within medicine that they could work. The principal focus of their use, to relieve the pain of surgical interventions, seemed to most practitioners fanciful and illusionary conjecture. Pain and cutting into the body seemed inseparable events. Disbelief in the possibility of anesthetic therapy, thus, led practitioners to be skeptical about reports of achieving the goal. Patients who underwent operations and experienced unmitigated suffering and the surgeons performing it could take no other realistic position. So claims made by scientists such as the British chemist Sir Humphry Davy in the late eighteenth century of the power of nitrous oxide to render people insensitive to pain were viewed skeptically and dismissed. But as exploration of substances with anesthetic properties grew, skepticism lessened and the door was open for a convincing trial.

The event that proved the reality of anesthesia was a surgical test conducted in an amphitheater at Massachusetts General Hospital on October 16, 1846, before an audience of surgeons and medical students. Twenty-seven-year-old Gilbert Abbott, a patient with a vascular tumor of the neck, was to be given ether by a dentist, William T. G.

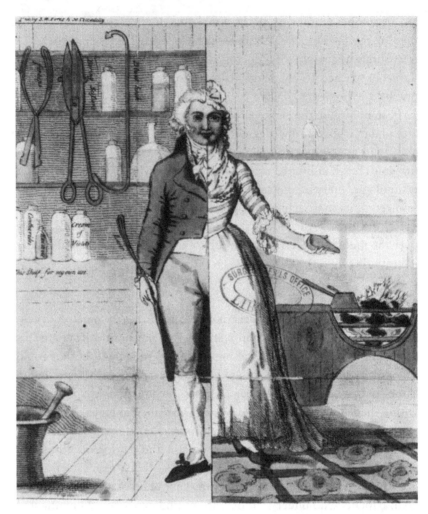

Figure 20. A hybrid portrayal of male and female birthing practitioners. It is a visual play on the term *man-midwife*, the name given to male surgeons and physicians in the seventeenth century who began to attend births. Other descriptors denoting a birth attendant and preferred by male practitioners was the French term *accoucheur*; or the title *obstetrician*, derived from the Latin word for "midwife," *obstetrix*. In the illustration, the man is surrounded by drugs and potions, as well as instruments, one of which he has in his hand. The woman holds only a papboat used to feed babies, and the scene behind her is of a home with a comforting hearth. It is meant to contrast a technologically driven versus a humanistically centered approach to childbirth. Frontispiece from S. W. Fore's *Man-Midwifery Dissected*... London, 1795. Courtesy of the National Library of Medicine.

Morton, who had investigated and confirmed its anesthetic properties in his practice. Newspaper accounts of his work had led Dr. John
Collins Warren, a well-known surgeon practicing at the hospital, to
invite him to administer the pain-relieving preparation, whose nature
Morton had kept secret. The time for the operation arrived but Morton
had not. An impatient Warren began preparations to proceed. But as
Abbott was being strapped in the operating chair, Morton appeared,
late from tinkering with his equipment. He connected the patient to a
glass globe containing the anesthetic and from which Abbott breathed
in the pain-killing vapor. What happened next is described by Morton's
wife: "Then in all parts of the amphitheatre there came a quick catching
of breath, followed by a silence almost deathlike, as Dr. Warren stepped
forward and prepared to operate.... The patient lay silent, with eyes
closed as if in sleep; but everyone present fully expected to hear a shriek
of agony ring out as the knife struck down into the sensitive nerves, but
the stroke came with no accompanying cry. Then another and another,
and still the patient lay silent, sleeping while the blood from the severed
artery spurted forth. The surgeon was doing his work, and the patient
was free from pain."

In thirty minutes the surgery ended, the patient awoke to confirm he
had felt no pain. Responding to this testimony Dr. Warren spoke to the
audience the now famous words: "'Gentlemen, this is no humbug.'"[17]

But when using the anesthetic liquid in a second operation was proposed by Warren to test whether it could still pain in a major operation –
in this case, amputation of a limb – opposition arose. The Massachusetts
Medical Society opposed the participation of doctors in a trial and clinical use of a secret remedy. Its stand reflected a growing concern for the
ethical aspects of practice during the nineteenth century, undergirded by
the seminal and influential 1803 work of the English physician Thomas
Percival, *Medical Ethics*. In it, he asserted: "No Physician or Surgeon
should dispense a secret nostrum, whether it be his invention, or exclu-
sive property; for, if it be of real efficacy, the concealment of it is
inconsistent with beneficence and professional liberality; and if mystery
alone give it value and importance, such craft implies either disgraceful
ignorance or fraudulent avarice."[18]

Minutes before the operation was to proceed, with or without
Morton, he relented and revealed that his anesthetic was sulphuric ether.
He could not bear to see the patient suffer when he had the power to

prevent it. Humaneness had vanquished self-interest. Veils over significant discoveries, such as that which the Chamberlens had placed over the obstetric forceps, were being lifted in a medical environment becoming more ethically minded.

The success of ether opened the gates of inquiry to identify other anesthetic agents. And in childbirth more were needed. While ether was quickly adopted to meliorate the suffering of labor, it sometimes produced disturbing side effects such as irritating the bronchi of the lungs, a sharp and pungent smell; and further, large amounts of time and anesthetic were needed to produce and maintain pain relief. These issues led the English physician and obstetrician James Y. Simpson to search for an alternative substance with fewer problems. He discovered one on November 4, 1847. Sitting at a table in his house with two colleagues, he sampled and found that chloroform was a potent anesthetic. He administered it successfully four days later to a colleague's wife in labor, who in gratitude named her baby girl Anaesthesia.[19]

A great burden for pregnant women was anticipating the suffering unleashed during the experience of birth. Thus, women embraced, and even demanded, anesthetic agents that offered relief from such anguish. One was Fanny Longfellow, wife of the poet Henry Wadsworth Longfellow. On April 7, 1847, she became the first woman in the United States to request and receive ether during childbirth. She was attended by Nathan Cooley Keep, a physician and dean of dentistry at Harvard, who had used it in dental surgery and had designed an apparatus to deliver it, from which Fanny inhaled. "The sufferings of her last moments were greatly mitigated," her husband Henry reported. Fanny, who bore a girl, was delighted, as she described in a letter to her sister-in-law: "I am very sorry you all thought me so rash and naughty in trying the ether. Henry's faith gave me courage and I had heard such a thing had succeeded abroad, where the surgeons extend this great blessing much more boldly and universally than our timid doctors. . . . This is certainly the greatest blessing of this age and I am glad to have lived at the time of its coming and in the country which gives it to the world."[20]

Unlike its use in surgery, where total pain relief that rendered patients unconscious was called for, during birth anesthesia was kept moderate to enlist the mother's efforts in expelling the baby. Still, many physicians opposed its use in childbirth out of concern for lessening the force of the woman's natural contractions and fears about its safeness, for it was hazardous in inexperienced hands. What is more, the insensitivity and loss of consciousness it could produce appeared uncomfortably similar to the appearance of death.

However, before these anesthetics could achieve widespread use, they had to confront a formidable obstacle that had nothing to do with medicine. The barrier was erected by religious institutions and the rationale for putting it up was biblical. Some clergy and doctors as well believed that the declaration in Genesis 3:16 imposing painful childbirth as a punishment for Eve's sin in the Garden of Eden required physicians to refrain from using anesthesia. A particularly heated theological and medical debate on this issue took place in England and was resolved in 1853, when Dr. John Snow successfully used chloroform for the birth of the eighth child of Queen Victoria. Fittingly when its discoverer James Y. Simpson was given the royal title of baronet in 1866, he chose for the inscription on his coat of arms *Victo dolore*, pain conquered.[21]

The decision to use anesthesia in childbirth is described by a Virginia practitioner writing in 1884:

I came into practice just when the God-given boon had been first used and commended to the world.... I heard it denounced by a distinguished and revered preceptor as dangerous, cruel, and a criminal contravention of the Divine curse: "In sorrow shalt thou bring forth children."... And though I used it at as early a date as any of my compeers, I used it for a time only in bad cases, and I used it hesitatingly – and as it were under protest – accepting it as an evil.... Since then I have learned to accept it as a boon – a benefaction beyond all computation, and now I believe that the conditions and circumstances should be very rare and very peculiar which would justify a practitioner in withholding its blessing from a woman in the agony of childbirth. Nothing gives me so much pleasure as the promise of that Lethe ["oblivion," from Greek myth] to the expectant mother when the fearful hour draws nigh, except the fulfillment of that promise, and her grateful expression of returning consciousness – "Is it indeed all over, and is my baby born?"

Accordingly, during the second half of the nineteenth century, the particular experiences with anesthesia of individual patients and doctors dictated its embrace. But by the century's end, ether or chloroform was used in about half of medically attended births.[22]

Relieving the pain of childbirth, however, had no effect on subduing one of its major hazards – puerperal (meaning "afterbirth") fever, which threatened the lives of mothers following delivery. At this time, while physicians thought a given disease could have multiple causes, following a Hippocratic perspective they considered environmental factors most significant. "Matter floating in the air" was the phrase used by the eminent eighteenth-century doctor William Cullen to characterize these factors. Infectious inanimate matter could arise from swampy ground or urban filth and create illnesses in the general population, such as malaria (bad air). Patients could generate it also and cause epidemics within the confined space of a hospital. And it was in the lying-in hospital, an observer wrote in 1848, that puerperal fever found its "greatest perfection."[23]

Making ordinary hospitals a center of childbirth and, in the mid-eighteenth century, founding lying-in hospitals mainly to serve the birthing needs of the poor were developments that reflected the growing popularity of having physicians and surgeons deliver babies. It is ironic that their educational and research needs, scope of practice, and theoretical beliefs strongly contributed to the rising incidence of puerperal fever in the nineteenth century. Physicians and surgeons who had rejected obstetric practice as professionally diminishing and a diversion from their usual duties were given unique opportunities in the hospital to study the disorders of pregnancy and birth. In their wards they could follow the progression of symptoms in puerperal fever and other diseases, and at the autopsy table view the lesions producing the patient's suffering. And they used this learning to institute better care. However, physicians and surgeons brought hospitalized pregnant women not only scientific know-how but also exposure to diseases encountered in practice and explored during autopsy. Still, practitioners did not believe the routines of medical life threatened birthing patients. The prevailing theory on how disease spread focused on an atmospheric transmission and did not suggest the possibility of a person-to-person route.

In the late eighteenth century and well into the nineteenth century, physicians who sought to explain and vanquish puerperal fever challenged this enshrined theoretical perspective. And their explanations involved as causal factors not only infectious hospital environments but surgeons and doctors themselves. This last connection was forcibly argued in a 1795 treatise by the Scottish surgeon Alexander Gordon, who identified a relationship between puerperal fever and a common disease, erysipelas (both of which were later found to be caused by the same bacteria, streptococcus). But he also confessed: "It is a disagreeable declaration for me to mention, that I myself, was the means of carrying the infection to a great number of women."[24] In the nineteenth century an initially small chorus of medical opinion grew louder and more forceful in supporting the hypothesis of person-to-person spread of puerperal fever.

In the United States, the Harvard professor and eminent doctor Oliver Wendell Holmes argued the point tellingly in an 1843 essay. He described cases in which physicians who either cared for patients with puerperal fever or conducted autopsies on women who died from it, subsequently treated patients who got the disease. He cautioned the physicians in readiness to attend a birth to avoid performing autopsies of puerperal fever victims, and if merely an observer at one to "change every article of clothing" beforehand. Further, should a single case of the fever occur in his practice, the physician was "bound to consider the next female he attends in labor ... as in danger of being infected by him." In addition, three or more closely connected cases of the fever arising in a doctor's practice were to be taken as "*prima facie* evidence that he is the vehicle of contagion." And he declared, "the existence of a *private pestilence* in the sphere of a single physician should be looked upon not as a misfortune but a crime."[25]

Despite Holmes's clear recognition that the illness was generated by a yet-unknown contagion conveyed between individuals, like others of his time he believed that a given disease like puerperal fever had multiple causes, such as in this case polluting airborne matter. Other physicians proposed additional sources of puerperal fever, among which were mental instability, sedentary employment, and inadequate diet. Thus, in the mid-nineteenth century, although diseases were appreciated as separate entities distinguished by fingerprints they left on anatomical structures in the body and patterns of symptoms they generated in patients, nonetheless, when it came to the question of how they were delivered to people, the answer was – in many possible ways.

Achieving a specificity for the causes of diseases that matched the anatomical and symptomatical precision through which their uniqueness was established occurred later in the nineteenth century when the German physician Robert Koch and the French chemist Louis Pasteur, among others, demonstrated bacteria to be definitive disease-producing agents. However, in the interim, the concept of specific causation was proposed by a Hungarian physician whose work focused on puerperal fever, Ignaz Semmelweis. He forcefully argued against multiple causes of the disorder. Reasoning from the death in 1847 of his beloved teacher, Jakob Kolletschka, from a cut incurred while dissecting a corpse, and whose autopsy showed pathology similar to that found in women dying from puerperal fever, Semmelweis concluded that he and the women succumbed from the same disease and the same cause. Since it was clear that material from the corpse his teacher dissected had entered his body through the cut, Semmelweis concluded that decaying matter, introduced into the birth canal of women via the hands of physicians who carried it from autopsies or examinations conducted on other patients, was a basic and necessary cause of puerperal fever. He adopted chlorine washing by doctors to protect patients from this danger and reduced the mortality rate in his hospital clinic to about the 1 percent he regarded as optimal. Semmelweis thereby anticipated the concept that particular diseases had particular causes, which the imminent bacteriological era would definitively establish.[26]

Nearly two decades after Semmelweis began to publish his ideas (1848) and before the bacterial relationship to illness was established, using a line of reasoning similar to Semmelweis and confirmative of his work, Joseph Lister, professor of surgery at the Glasgow Royal Infirmary in Scotland, announced in 1867 the findings of a study on antisepsis. It was a crucial milestone not only for surgery but for all of medicine, including childbirth. Before Lister's work, surgical procedures carried great risk: in Britain during the 1860s, nearly half of patients who underwent major surgery died from wound infections attributed to unspecified contagions in the air, the prevailing view of the day. Lister, however, was attracted to the work of Pasteur, who was writing on the role of airborne organisms in spoiling milk and wine and, as noted, in producing diseases in humans. Lister theorized that perhaps such organisms entering the body through surgical openings might thereby infect it. As Humphreys noted: "While Pasteur destroyed germs by heat, Lister concentrated on cleanliness. He washed his hands frequently and insisted on laundered towels. Using carbolic acid as an agent of antisepsis, he sterilized his instruments, soaked wound dressings, and sprayed the substance liberally around the operating area."[27] Using the technique over a period of almost two years, Lister treated the wounds caused by compound fractures of the leg in eleven patients and described the results in a series of reports published in the *Lancet* during 1867. At that time, the treatment for infection and the deadly gangrene it produced, the result of compound fractures generally, was amputation of the leg – a procedure that carried an almost 50 percent mortality. But in Lister's series, ten patients recovered uneventfully and only one died.[28]

This unheard-of success rate established antiseptic procedure as an essential part of surgery and affirmed its usefulness in other parts of medicine, including childbirth. When in 1869 Pasteur demonstrated the association of the streptococcus bacteria and puerperal fever, he gave tangible form to the anonymous airborne contagions against which Lister had directed his antiseptic agent and provided a scientific grounding for the experimental evidence that formed the basis of antiseptic use. A year later, the Swiss obstetrician Johann Bischoff, who had visited Lister's Glasgow hospital and witnessed the results of his antiseptic procedure, was applying the antiseptic method of Lister to reduce puerperal fever deaths in his hospital. By the 1880s most American and British lying-in hospitals had adopted the technique, with dramatic success. In England, before 1880 maternal mortality in lying-in hospitals was more than two hundred deaths per ten thousand births. After 1880 maternal mortality fell to twenty or less.[29]

Whether this reduction in maternal mortality was achievable in the home, where around the turn of the twentieth century about nine out of ten births occurred, would rest on the ability of practitioners to use the technologies of mortality-reduction effectively there. And this was a major problem. Antiseptic techniques were often applied halfheartedly in home settings, as both birthing mothers and doctors were stifled by the rigors of implementing the tedious measures required to use them properly. Further, the physical environment and family personalities of every home as well as the practice habits, temperament, and medical beliefs of every doctor were different, and this combination created a large unpredictability in the outcome of care. Ironically, these problems worsened as advances were made in achieving greater protection against microbial infection. By the late nineteenth century, the concept of antisepsis, directed at killing bacteria already in place, was replaced by the notion of asepsis – an effort to prevent bacterial contamination in the first place. Aseptic measures such as the use of rubber gloves, sterile sheets, and shaving hair around surgical sites were measures that increased the safeness of medical interventions.

But efforts to implement these aseptic measures were even more difficult than were the antiseptic ones in diverse home environments that never were intended to be sterile settings, and with family members, including the birthing woman, viewing homes as castles in which they reigned supreme. A physician cautioned colleagues of the risk of attempting the aseptic measure of shaving the pubic hair of a woman in labor: "In about three seconds after the doctor has made the first rake with his safety [razor], he will find himself on his back out in the yard with the imprint of a woman's bare foot emblazoned on his manly chest, the window sash around his neck and a revolving vision of all the stars in the firmament presented to him. Tell him not to try to shave 'em."[30]

In the face of problems that thwarted effective application of birthing technologies in the home, a transformative solution beckoned – change the site of care. The effectiveness of virtually every sector of medicine had risen during the nineteenth century as a result of new technologies and concepts of disease transmission, which by the end of the century gave an old and troubled institution, the hospital, a new and crucial role in bringing to patients and doctors the fruits of medicine's scientific developments. For childbirth as well as for disease, the nineteenth-century hospital had been a dangerous place to be, shunned by all who could afford to have medical care in the home because of the epidemics of life-threatening infection that spread continually within its walls. Made relatively safe and offering advantages essential to practicing technological medicine, in the twentieth century the hospital became the center of care.

The transition from home to hospital for childbirth is displayed in the case records of the New York Lying-In Hospital's Outdoor Department on Broome Street in New York City. They reveal the work and experiences of patients and staff in this new setting of care.[31] Created in 1890, over the next forty-one years the facility delivered home-based obstetrical services to almost fifty thousand women on the city's Lower East Side through a staff headed by leading obstetricians. The main clients were Jewish working-class immigrants whose compliance with physician directives and student education needs were preconditions for acceptance. This raised problems. Midwives sharing the immigrants' language and gender and having their respect were available and sought by them to assist with birth. But physicians believed that the midwives endangered women and affronted their professional dignity when seeking to join them in attending deliveries. And on this subject Outdoor Department policy was rigid: a choice was required between physician- and midwife-assisted birth. Though women wished it, they could not have both.

Another matter troubled pregnant women: they disliked the frequent examinations to follow labor made by doctors and students. For the latter, dilation of the cervical opening of the uterus to at least three-finger breadths marked its true medical beginning. So cases of strongly felt uterine contractions but inadequate cervical dilation were labeled by doctors as "false" labor. Pregnant women did not discount these subjective feelings and resented their significance belittled. The women also disliked restrictions such as limits placed on their activities after birth, but they faced dismissal from care if they were not followed. This outcome is reflected in a terse medical note: "Patient up working – cooking – and complained of some pains but said she must work. Discharged."[32]

Reflecting obstetric practice at this time of transition between home and hospital birth, department physicians unrealistically insisted that home delivery share the scientific standards that hospitals imposed on birth. As Dye observed: "Unlike the typical nineteenth century practitioner, anxious to please his patient and her family by accommodating himself to cultural standards of decorum and popular birthing customs, the Broome Street doctors consciously worked to systematize obstetrics and to integrate scientific knowledge with everyday practice."[33] Thus, the Outdoor Department, as an arm of the hospital, extended its body of learning and authority into the home. It demanded that the physician's word reign in deciding who should be part of the birth process, what signs of birth progress were noteworthy, what interventions were needed, and how the recovery period should be managed. In asserting their authority, doctors placed the requirements of scientific medicine above the need for human understanding.

Women accepted this hegemony and focus to secure the health of themselves and their babies. But gradually the department's role declined, its status as a way station between home and hospital care affirmed when J. P. Morgan replaced the old lying-in hospital with a million-dollar structure opened in 1902. Then 2,619 births were outpatient deliveries and 725 inpatient ones, a ratio of about three to one babies born at home. In 1906 the ratio was three to two; in 1914 it evened; and it became in 1918 three to two in the hospital's favor.[34]

But at this time, a cloud hovered over childbirth. The decline in maternal mortality at leading lying-in hospitals around the world after the introduction of aseptic techniques in the 1880s was not followed by an overall decrease at a national level in all Western countries. This was most notable in Britain and the United States, where professional incompetence, poor aseptic technique, and overuse of technology in normal labor in both home and hospital deliveries were blamed. This problem was depicted in a stern warning given to doctors in 1902 by the editors of the *Journal of the American Medical Association*:

The physician feels that if he is aseptic in his work...he can do practically what he will. The old rule of "meddlesome midwifery is bad" is cast aside. With improved forceps of several patterns, with chloroform given with practically no danger, even the careful physician feels justified in early instrumental interference, resorts to version on slight provocation, is indifferent to lacerations because he can sew them up immediately, is digitally diligent in determining the progress of labor; in fact, he hesitates at none of these because he has practically no fear of sepsis. And why? Because by his side is a bowl of bichloride solution or of carbolic acid or of some other favorite antiseptic into which he dips his fingers, his silk, his forceps, perhaps, flattering himself that in this way he is rendering himself clean and protecting his patient from harm.... There is a slip somewhere in the technique of his asepsis and the deed is done.... These tragedies are occurring every day...a careless obstetrician, over-confident because of his fancied protection by his so-called asepsis, may be a breeder of the most serious mischief.[35]

The presence of these technologies created increasing incentives to intervention in childbirth. The same diagnosis was made in a 1936 talk in the United States by the English obstetrician James Young. He described the practices of many British and American doctors as an "orgy of interference" and blamed the existing high maternal mortality rate on unacceptable antiseptic practices, excessive medical interventions, and inadequate obstetric education. But at this mid-1930s time, a remarkable change occurred: maternal mortality began to fall in England, the United States, and around the Western world. The

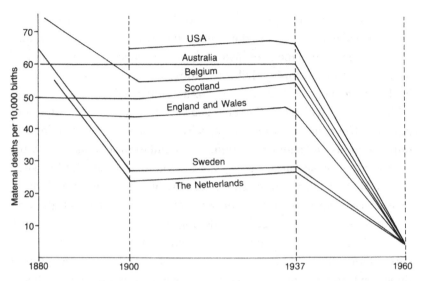

Figure 21. Maternal mortality trends, 1880–1960 (In Loudon ISL. Childbirth. In WF Bynum and R Porter (eds.), *Companion Encyclopedia of the History of Medicine*. London: Routledge; 1993, 1059).

immediate cause was the introduction of a sulfonamide drug, Prontsil, that attacked the bacterial source of puerperal fever, the streptococcus, virtually eliminating the most common cause of maternal deaths. Further, investigators discovered that this organism inhabited the nose and throat of healthy people. Thus, in a throwback to the nineteenth century, medical practitioners again could be unwitting sources of infection. Not only carefully following other aspects of asepsis but wearing surgical masks as well now became essential during birth attendance.[36] These advances were followed by the improvement of obstetric education and hospital services, among other things. By 1960 maternal mortality in Western countries had declined to uniformly low levels (Figure 21), and in the United States almost all births now occurred in hospitals, a situation that has prevailed to the present.[37] But this time was not only a terminus of biologically transformative alteration of childbirth – it also marked the beginning of equally significant changes in its social dimensions.

The arrangements of authority and care that governed the relationship between doctors and patients in general and pregnant women especially, in all settings of care from the home to the hospital, were irrevocably transformed in the decade of the 1960s, one of the most tumultuous and creative periods in American history. It was marked by a confluence of four momentous events: a civil rights movement, a women's rights and health movement, an antiwar and counterculture ethos, and a medical ethics renewal, which together changed social values, relationships, and policies. The civil rights movement stirred Americans to examine not only the rights and standing of minority populations but also the status of individuals in significant relationships bounding American life, such as government with citizen, employer with worker, parent and child, professor and student, and doctor with patient. The women's rights and health movement challenged the ideologies that restricted sovereignty over self and the status and role of women in society and in health-care relationships. These changes were reinforced by a counterculture movement among the young, largely in reaction against the war being fought in Vietnam, which caused them to question and flout social conventions and expectations and to live with mores and goals different from those of their parents. And a medical ethics renewal challenged the current values of medical practice by producing a new set of rights for patients anchored in autonomy – the right of the individual to be self-governing in all aspects of life, including health care. The energies released by these events produced a social and ethical tide that lifted the aspirations of all who lived in relationships that limited their rights and freedom.

This reformist spirit in American culture catalyzed a major change in society and its response to medicine: the assertion by health consumers and patients of a right to be self-governing in their personal interactions with medicine and a determination to learn more about medicine and improve the system that delivered its care. A crucial organization formed at the beginning of the modern consumer health movement and pivotal to its identity and success was the Boston Women's Health Book Collective. Its founding participants, who began weekly meetings in Boston at the end of the 1960s, were among the early groups of women in other parts of the country who gathered to share health-care experiences, explore how they were treated by the American medical-care system, and produce health information focused on the needs of women. To spread its ideals, the collective developed a course for women on health, sexuality, and childbearing. As a participant in these activities wrote: "In recounting our life stories and health care experiences, we discovered with surprise and elation that the 'personal is political' – that we were not alone in what happened to us. By pooling all we knew about ourselves, we could create a useful body of knowledge. We soon realized that forces much larger than ourselves determined the availability and quality of health and medical care, and that by working in unison and sharing our knowledge and clout, we could become a force to alter the system to meet our needs."[38]

A major outcome of this effort, the 1970 book *Our Bodies, Ourselves*, was crucial in starting and maintaining the women's health movement nationally and internationally. By the century's end it had sold some 4 million copies worldwide. From its first to its later editions, the work summarized the experiences of hundreds of women as it examined medicalization of the bodies and lives of women, meshed holistic and conventional medical knowledge, and located the personal medical experiences of women in a sociopolitical context that transcended the more individually-centered approach that was the focus of traditional self-help groups. It explored the search for and maintenance of women's health in the context of sexism and racism and condemned the corporate structure and philosophy of the medical establishment and its financial and profit-driven nature. It challenged women to share experiences and acquire knowledge to question the assumptions underlying received care, to better not only their own health but the American medical system as well. "Our illness is our business," wrote an early member of the women's health movement, summing up a key purpose. And this ideal was tied by her to another goal – change – which started with the individual and then spread to the community.[39]

Childbearing has remained a central focus in *Our Bodies, Ourselves*. Its 1998 edition states: "We bring to childbirth our histories, our relationships, our rituals, our needs and values that relate to intimacy, our sexuality, the quality and style of family life and community, and our deepest beliefs about life, birth and death."[40] The work continues to reinforce the historical ideals of the women's health movement in its focus on respecting the identity and wishes of women, the naturalness of birth, the dangers of making it too medical, and the significance of birth's cultural and social context. There is a strong emphasis on women listening to their bodies and trusting in the normality of birth, and the benefits of attendance by practitioners affirming these values and creating a *"climate of confidence,"* which inspires women to shape their own birthing experience. This is contrasted with the *"climate of doubt,"* worry, and fear, which it declared had historically dominated American obstetric practice and could be largely attributed to medicine's technological appetite.

The additional problem that this technology was controlled by a male-dominated health profession, which left inadequate room for female midwives to practice more widely, evoked much concern in the women's health movement, as did the placing of birth in the hospital:

"Women experience the influence of the hospital setting long before labor begins. With the increasing routine use of pregnancy screening procedures, we are visiting hospitals earlier and earlier. When we enter these places for sick people, it is difficult not to view pregnancy, birth, and our bodies as unhealthy.... As we become "patients" and our experience is defined in medical terms, we become part of an impersonal production process. Upon entering the hospital in labor, we are often placed in wheelchairs. Our personal effects are removed. We are among strangers. We become anonymous. We are immobilized, hooked up to fetal monitors and IVs. Each "stage" of labor is allotted a certain amount of time, and no more.... Such hospital routines debilitate us. We become passive, dependent."[41,42]

The women's health movement set out to alter the environment, philosophy, and practices of birth. And energized by their ideas and work, childbearing and birthing practices in America began to change. Women started to question the need for strict hospital routines based on scientific measures carried too far that ignored social and personal needs. Prominent among them was a concern by hospitals to maintain a strict aseptic environment during and after birth to prevent infection. It resulted in excluding fathers from the delivery room, and after birth separating mothers from babies by confining them to nurseries. Family visits to see newborns meant viewing them through a nursery window. The new ethos led parents to successfully challenge such measures.

It also stimulated their interest in natural childbirth, which excluded sedation by drugs, emphasized relaxation techniques for pain and discomfort, and advocated education to prepare for the events of pregnancy and birth. These ideas had been proposed earlier by pioneers such as Grantly Dick-Read, in his 1944 book *Childbirth without Fear: The Principles and Practice of Natural Childbirth*, and Ferdinand Lamaze, a French doctor whose work was brought to American attention by

Marjorie Karmel's 1959 book *Thank You, Dr. Lamaze*. Karmel related the benefits of the unmedicated birth experience she had in France and the problems of having a medicated labor in America. Thus, in the 1970s classes for expectant mothers appeared based on the natural birth ideas proposed by Read and techniques to achieve it developed by Lamaze. The classes were meant not only to instruct expectant women but also to educate fathers to be an assistant and a nurturing presence at birth. To have this role required families to overcome hospital concerns: Would fathers contaminate sterile environments? Tolerate the sight of suffering? Be repelled by the blood of birth?[43] Informed families dispelled these concerns and gradually began to moderate other kinds of hospital resistance to change.

As noted earlier, the trend to hospital birth that began in the twentieth century has continued to the present, with almost all births in the United States occurring there.[44] But the diffusion of medical knowledge to create a variety of safe environments for birth, within as well as outside of hospitals, and a public growing more educated about it, have increasingly freed women and their partners to choose the birthing experience and venue they wish, and also to view childbirth more as a natural human event than as a problematic medical condition.

Throughout the past four centuries, the development of technologies to treat the experience of birth has separated and diminished the significance of its social, cultural, and personal aspects, from a quest to ensure the physical safety of mother and child. We explore in the next and concluding chapter just how such a separation is produced by technology, in birth and in other aspects of health care, and we examine its nature and governance.

9

GOVERNING THE EMPIRE
OF MACHINES

When Thomas Sydenham proposed in the seventeenth century that diseases were like plants, discrete and tangible entities having distinctive characteristics, he helped establish a way of thinking that would transform medicine. To do this, the reader will recall, he stripped disease entities down to their essence. And this, he reasoned, required excising from them symptoms that expressed the patient's uniqueness but retaining ones commonly held by the population having the disease. The process removed from medical consideration personality-based evidence confusing to and therefore according to this logic unnecessary in the diagnosis of a disease.

Sydenham's separation of symptoms to sculpt disease categories was, essentially, the same action G. B. Morgagni took in the eighteenth century. He dissected corpses to locate, hiding amid their normal tissue, the pathological structural changes that both generated symptoms in living patients and, by their specific appearance at autopsy, revealed the diseases they had. Both Sydenham and Morgagni engaged in the practice of analysis, the separation of wholes into parts to identify diseases. And this approach nourished the soil from which sprang modern medical technology.

In general, technologies are created by the existence of possibilities that the prevailing ideas, culture, and social climate of an era suggest to an innovator could be useful, interesting, or profitable. Thus, technologies are absorptive and reflective: they soak up and mirror back aspects of the environment in which they are created. In medicine, the prevailing theoretical climate is a powerful influence on this creative process.

Technological innovations are typically made to extend and increase the power of a dominant theory, which in nineteenth-century medicine was analytically based anatomical thinking.

The first major technological expression of anatomical thinking in medicine came from Laennec in the early part of that century, when he invented the stethoscope. It detected in the living patient physical signs of interior anatomical disruptions, which allowed doctors to dissect the body to locate diseases without piercing its skin. Thus, the stethoscope was as much an instrument of anatomical analysis as the scalpel. Its clinical use, along with other instruments performing in a like manner on other parts of the body, introduced this type of thinking into the diagnostic arena of practice.

In the twentieth century, anatomical thinking became firmly established in the therapeutic part of medicine. Efforts to create specific treatments for specific diseases accelerated, largely directed at the bacteria newly associated with their cause. Paul Ehrlich, who in 1907 discovered Salvarsan, an arsenic-based drug with a direct effect on the bacterial organism causing the widespread disease syphilis, also coined a phrase that would resonate in subsequent therapeutic investigations throughout the twentieth century: "magic bullet." By this, he meant that an ideal therapy directed its actions to only the desired area or entity of pathology, harming no other tissues en route to its mission. Such therapy, in other words, had lesion specificity. The therapy sought the place of pathology in the same way as the scalpel or stethoscope did when they were deployed to treat or identify a disease. In each case, anatomical thinking was present and compelling.

The theoretical mind-set of anatomical thinking reinforced another generic characteristic of technologies – focus. Technologies are material inventions developed to extend or replace human capabilities. They have two essential dimensions: form and purpose. Their form is designed to most effectively carry out their purpose. Thus, a round wooden tube having a bore through its center was the form Laennec decided was best suited for the purpose of auscultation, evaluating the sounds generated within the body. Technology changes as new forms are devised to better fulfill purpose or as the purpose itself is expanded or limited. The hold of technologies on us is their power to channel our attention to those aspects of reality they were designed to influence and portray: they are directive. Powerful technologies, by definition, draw us into defined spaces with a riveting intensity, shutting out surrounding realities to enhance the importance of the action or place to which they take us. In sum, absorptive, reflective, and directive characteristics are critical features of technologies. In the process of creating them, inventors tune into the spirit of their time and integrate aspects of it into their innovations. Users, in turn, are channeled toward the actions and thinking embedded in the innovation.

The advantage conferred by the ability of technologies to act with such focused intensity is purchased at a price – tuning out and diminishing the significance of other aspects of reality. This has important consequences for medical care. Particularly critical has been withdrawal of attention from personal, cultural, and social expressions of illness by technologies designed to explore or treat its physical aspects. An example from the previous discussion of childbirth is decreased attention to the personal needs of the mother and the cultural associations and meanings of birth to families and communities, as technologies were introduced to increase birth's biological safety. The focus on this latter and clearly important purpose was so intense that it was as if social and psychological needs lacked significance. Medical attendants increasingly introduced technological agents into birth – forceps, surgical tools, anesthesia, antisepsis, and so forth – which directed attention to its physical aspects. This was followed by removing birth from the home and placing it in the doctor's workshop – the hospital – where attention to its physical aspects could be undertaken with a greater intensity. The example reflects the convergence of anatomical thinking and technological focus – a centuries-old merger that continues to pervade contemporary medicine and create problems for it. For while this fractionation of wholes produces powerful agents of cure, it spawns powerful disincentives to care. Humanistically, the subject of care is the person, who cannot be understood fully if divided into parts by the thinking and technology of medicine.

A basic issue for contemporary American society is how to bring the technological and humanistic features of medicine into balance. The consumer health movement, for which the women's health movement was a major impetus, is an important force in attaining this goal. And greatly supporting the concerns that draw consumers to this effort – a rising expectation from care, a rising understanding of care, and a rising interest in changing care – is the power of information. Consumers acquire health information through two basic sources: from doctors as their patients and from social institutions (including medicine) as members of the public. We explore first the contributions of doctors to this development.

Information about the workings of the body and therapies to improve and heal it has always been the essential coin of the medical realm, and physicians themselves have been vitally concerned about the conditions for giving it out. An early expression of this is found in the profoundly significant 2,500-year-old Hippocratic oath.[1] It declares that would-be students could not receive a medical education unless first committing themselves to the oath's ethical principles. In this way, the Greek oath swearing was different from the ones now used, which occur after acceptance to or upon graduation from medical school rather than before admission to it. Why? Because the Greeks were exceedingly cautious about disclosing medicine's knowledge. They would not entrust it to those who had not first made a commitment to use the knowledge in accordance with revered practice values, especially ones that served the interest of the patient rather than the interest of the self.

The Greeks considered the conditions of giving and withholding information not only in matters of education but also in matters of patient care. They believed in the doctor's responsibility to protect patients from misgivings, anxieties, and decline, and this extended to withholding foreboding facts from them. As trustees and implementers of medical knowledge, Greek physicians understood the profound influence their comments could have on the patient's physical and mental state. They recognized that the doctor's words could wound as deeply as the surgeon's blade and developed a cautionary view of their use. No passage in the Hippocratic works describes this better than one from *Decorum*: "Perform [therapies] calmly and adroitly, concealing most things from the patient while you are attending to him. Give necessary orders with cheerfulness and serenity, turning his attention away from what is being done to him; sometimes reprove sharply and emphatically, and sometimes comfort with solicitude and attention, revealing nothing of the patient's future or present condition. For many patients through this cause have taken a turn for the worse, I mean by the declaration I have mentioned of what is present, or by a forecast of what is to come."[2]

The advice given in this passage reflects insight into the power of emotions to heal or injure. Greek physicians understood the necessity of turning emotional forces in a positive direction, particularly in cases of grave illness, which meant enveloping patients in an atmosphere of hope. Achieving this state required deception, an action justified by the countervailing weight of the directive to benefit patients, a central ethic in Hippocratic medicine. Thus, by withholding information from patients, Greek doctors reasoned that they prevented harm and provided help.

Remarkably, the counsel in *Decorum* to cloud the true condition of patients as a means to sustain hope and secure recovery was referred to and restated as standard medical doctrine to the mid-twentieth century, a longevity of more than two millennia. Its last vestige is documented in a 1961 survey of more than two hundred Chicago physicians. Responding to the issue of what they told patients having cancer about their disease, almost 90 percent said they withheld this information. However, all survey participants shared the knowledge with a family member as a substitute for disclosure to patients. The rationale for withholding the cancer diagnosis from patients all converged, as the study's author writes, "to a single major goal: maintenance of hope. No inference was necessary to elicit this finding. Every single physician interviewed spontaneously emphasized this point and indicated his resolute and determined purpose is to sustain and bolster the patient's hope. Each in his own way communicates the possibility, even the likelihood, of recovery.... The modal policy is to tell as little as possible in the most general terms consistent with maintaining cooperation in treatment."[3]

During the 1960s and 1970s, sociologists and physicians began to study other reasons for doctors' withholding of information from patients, and how they justified prolonging the uncertainty and anxiety of patients by a decision to be silent about what they knew about their illness. This was done not only in cases of disease likely to be fatal but also in other serious conditions that were not, and even in situations in which patients were on their way to recovery. Extending a theory used in sociology to study behavior in bureaucracy, Waitzkin and Stoeckle, well known for their studies of doctor-patient interactions, concluded:

"The physician enhances his power to the extent that he can maintain the patient's uncertainty about the course of illness, efficacy of therapy, or specific future actions of the physician himself."[4]

Nevertheless, doctors gradually relinquished their hold on patient information, moved by the force of the rights movements of the 1960s and the exploration of disclosure by health professionals and institutions. The publication in 1973 by the American Hospital Association (AHA) of the Patient's Bill of Rights was a significant mark of this shift.[5] It asserts rights for patients through twelve principles, each of which begins with the phrase "The patient has the right to... " It thus views these rights not as entitlements given to patients by hospitals or physicians but as ones they hold inherently as individuals. The AHA statement also takes a large step forward through its focus, in three of the twelve principles, on giving patients rights to information. Patients would be informed about the risks and benefits of treatment, when changes to care were instituted, what other medical alternatives they had, the affiliations and relationships of the hospital and its professional staff with other health institutions, and their diagnosis and prognosis.

In the 1970s further research on disclosure revealed the flaws of prior medical thinking on the subject. Patients given information about what was wrong and what might happen to them were more hopeful than those not given such facts.[6] Informed patients had a clear interpretation of their illness and could anticipate not only the bad things that might happen but also the good. Indeed, prior generations of doctors who worried about disclosure were under the illusion that they could successfully conceal the perils of dire illness from their patients. They were wrong. People recognize when they are in danger. Symptoms that persist and are debilitating and unresponsive to therapy alert people to the fact that their problem is serious. Familiarity with disorders from which other family or community members suffered, or in more modern times from what they learned from public media, gave patients additional grounds through which to discern their peril. But the climate of denial that illness existed, created not only by doctors but also by family and friends who were inducted into a medical cover-up, left the patient alone, unable to share anxieties or suspicions about the true state of things. Thus, tragically, this policy of concealing information resulted in isolating patients from those they trusted most at a time when they were needed most. For these reasons, the new policy of openness to information was a great step forward in the care of patients. The most recent twenty-first-century expression of this openness is the growing establishment of personal health records by patients, with the cooperation of medical practitioners and institutions (see Chapter 5).

Historically, just as doctors limited information transmitted in the clinical relationship, they did the same about disseminating medical knowledge to the public. Until the seventeenth century medical books were widely written in Latin, a language that restricted access to their contents to the learned. Thereafter, they were increasingly composed in vernacular languages. Still, their technical complexity eluded public understanding. Although treatises and essays on preserving health and treating illness were published for the laity, by physicians as well as others, generally they did not adequately expose the public to the scientific debates, controversies, and theoretical complexities that pervaded professional literature.

Such forays by the public into the inner world of medicine grew in the twentieth century. But even in the period up through midcentury, some medical libraries, mainly driven by the physicians who helped govern them, restricted the access of consumers and patients to the works within them: the libraries worried about potential harms resulting from the misinterpretation and misuse of acquired knowledge when an untutored public encountered their works without professional guidance.[7] The policy regarding medical libraries thus repeated the cautionary approach to giving information found in medical relationships. Granted, information unaccompanied by understanding can injure as well as educate. But a policy of expanding the ability of public users to understand such information is preferable to restricting access to it. And in the 1960s such an expansion began. From that decade to the present, disclosures about the inner world of medicine have grown at a transformative pace, driven mainly by the movements of consumers to assert health-care rights, as the previous chapter discussed. In the past half century, numerous books written for consumers also appeared that demystified health-care science and treatment, described the hidden travails and encounters of students and residents as they studied medicine, and shared private journeys through illness and recovery, some written by doctors themselves. The latter works were especially poignant, for they often revealed surprise and consternation about the indignities suffered at the patient's end of the stethoscope or the surgeon's knife. Why, readers and reviewers asked, didn't their medical training give physicians the empathic skills to fathom patient feelings?

The consumer-oriented environment also generated a new spate of self-help groups, which emphasized "self-determination, self-reliance, self-production and self-empowerment," all directed at enhancing the internal resources of individuals.[8] A key aspect of the assistance they provided the public was information to cope with their problems and routes of communication to those who shared them. Many self-help groups were created, like ones that supported people having chronic illnesses from lupus to AIDS, helped patients and families cope with problems requiring long-term rehabilitative resources such as stroke and bereavement, provided knowledge for families and caregivers of the sick and disabled, and assisted people having addictions from drugs to gambling to navigate life without them. By 1990 more than 7 million Americans belonged to self-help groups. And at this time, a new technology that vastly enlarged public access to information and to one another, the Internet, was more than a decade old.

Given the name in 1982, the Internet originated as a U.S. Department of Defense project to study computer networking and facilitate collaboration among scientists living at different locations.[9] In the 1990s the Internet gained a significant place in personal and business life. It made communication virtually instantaneous, facilitated access to a voluminous and growing body of the world's knowledge, and permitted users to do this from any part of the globe at any time of day or night with a computer and an Internet connection. In one of the early major books to examine what the world of cyberspace meant to the world of health, the 1996 *Health Online*, the physician Tom Ferguson described ways people used this information universe:

I've found people reaching out for help – and others (very often the same people) reaching out *to* help. I've discovered a remarkable and impressive variety of new online support communities that have grown up spontaneously, with no publicity, no government planning, and no professional authorization. I've found people talking and sharing, exchanging information and support, listening and understanding each other: people in ones and twos and small groups and massive far-flung networks, people relating to each other – and to online health professionals – in startling and innovative new ways.

I learned that the information superhighway is not some vague vision just over the horizon. It's out there waiting for us right now. It's not much like a highway at all – more like a giant Brillo pad, with millions of self-helpers connected by modems and phone lines. Forget the 500-channel future. We're up to twenty million "channels" already and we're just getting warmed up.[10]

By the century's end, the nation also had a large and knowledgeable group of scholars, journalists, and filmmakers, as well as physicians and scientists, who provided the public with insights into the research, practice, and policies of medicine. The rise in the quality and volume of dependable public information about health care greatly bolstered public knowledge that was actionable to make personal decisions and shape social policies. Further, the increasing interest of the public in acquiring knowledge about the world of medicine led it to recognize a significant fact: that data generated by technology also carried significant social and cultural messages that had gone largely unnoticed by doctors. This development and its implications for medical practice are demonstrated in the evolution and use of ultrasound imaging to follow the growth of the fetus, which we now briefly examine.

Two calamitous events in the early twentieth century, a disaster at sea and a world war, catalyzed an interest in basic research on the generation of acoustic waves in seawater that ultimately led to ultrasound imaging. In 1912 a collision with an iceberg caused the *Titanic*, then the largest ship in the world, to sink on its maiden voyage. This led a British meteorologist to suggest the use of sound to locate submerged icebergs, an American engineer to establish its feasibility, and a French scientist in the midst of the First World War to invent a generator of high-frequency sound waves to detect submarines. When the waves hit a solid object and rebounded back to a monitor, if knowing the speed of sound, an object's distance and location could be determined. The device was extensively improved in the Second World War and called sonar (sound, navigation, and ranging technology). In the 1940s possible medical uses of ultrasound waves were explored: ultrasound images of the skull were made and its ability to screen women for lumps in the breast was investigated.[11]

In the following decade, the uterus became a subject of ultrasound through the pioneering work of the Scottish obstetrician Ian Donald after his appointment as a professor at the University of Glasgow in 1954. Military experience in the Second World War had familiarized Donald with sonar, and subsequent work in London introduced him to its medical possibilities. In 1957 Donald inadvertently made his first study of developing babies, when an ultrasound examination of a woman whose enlarged abdomen was clinically thought to be a fibroid revealed instead the head of a fetus. A year later, with colleagues, he published a watershed article in the *Lancet*, "Investigation of Abnormal Masses by Pulsed Ultrasound," which displayed images of a fetus's head, twins, an early pregnancy, and fibroids. Donald and other investigators of this period concluded from their scientific studies that, at the levels they used for diagnosis, ultrasound had no known harmful effects (Figure 22). This was a critical finding because before ultrasound, fetal development was followed with X-rays, whose use for this purpose ended in the 1950s when evidence of their danger to the fetus became overwhelming.[12] Later work confirmed the basic safeness of ultrasound.[13]

As the twentieth century ended, the use of ultrasound to evaluate fetal and maternal health had broadened to include assessing fetal age, growth, movement, and breathing; detecting multiple pregnancies; evaluating the structure and location of the placenta; screening for fetal abnormalities; and guiding instruments to sample fetal blood and uterine tissue as well as to carry out fetal therapy and surgery.[14] The fetus no longer "hides beneath our fingertips" or requires the doctor "to spend a lot of time guessing what is going on," wrote a physician. The technology had become "an active part in the management of pregnancy" with which one could observe the fetus, "visualize its motion, breathing, and activity, and bring reassurance to the mother" (Figure 23). As proof of ultrasound's value to doctors, patients, and society, by the mid-1990s some 250,000 machines existed in the world; about 250 million ultrasound examinations were done each year, largely for obstetric reasons; and Great Britain issued a commemorative stamp showing a mother and child alongside an ultrasound-generated fetal face (Figure 24).[15]

This account of ultrasound technology is gleaned from medical literature, in which its messages are presented as scientific data. However,

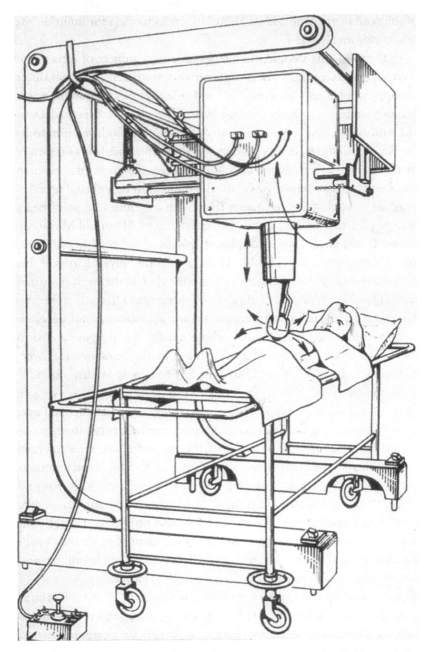

Figure 22. The automatic contact ultrasound scanner (1959). Reproduced with permission of the British Medical Ultrasound Society.

an alternative interpretation of ultrasound has been given, mainly by women, as an invention also sending significant cultural and social messages to which most physicians were not attuned.

As visual portrayal, ultrasound images share the characteristics of photographs, viewed alternatively in the history of photography as either objective statements or artistic representations. From its invention in the 1830s, and for more than a century thereafter, scientists and art critics agreed on photography's inherently objective nature. Scientists lauded their ability to capture with photography reality as it truly was. For the same reasons, art critics denounced photography as a technologically automated medium, lacking the subjective creativity of drawing and painting. Both were wrong. The photograph, from its taking to its production to its viewing, carries judgments and subjectiveness: bad for excessive scientific claims about it, good for artistic ones. Freed, then,

---

Figure 22 (*cont.*) This innovation replaced equipment first used by Donald for ultrasound imaging, which later commentators described as "large, unwieldy, unreliable, and messy," and whose pictures were "difficult to interpret and ridiculed by colleagues."[1] The new contact scanner was designed by Tom Brown, an engineer who in 1956 joined Donald's research team and credited him as "the real genius behind the massive technical development" of his group.[2] Brown was in charge not only of developing but also operating the new contact scanner in the clinic. He revealed that this assignment influenced his decision to automate the machine: "There was no way in which the Victorian establishment of the Western Infirmary, in the middle fifties, would ever countenance me, a young layman, laying hands directly on patients, especially gynaecological ones. Therefore, if I was going to take control of the examination conditions, I would have to use some other strategem. This was the real reason for developing the automatic scanner." Brown's design rationale reflects the basic historical problem of men examining women and is reminiscent of the problem facing Laennec in 1816 that led him to invent the stethoscope (see Chapter 1).

Brown goes on to describe the scanner's use: "The business end of this machine had a transducer mounted in a 'silver ball' reminiscent of the soap dispensers once common in public lavatories. It would walk its way across the surface of the abdomen, keeping a constant pressure, and rocking back and forwards through an angle of about plus and minus 30 degrees to the perpendicular to the skin, carrying out a thorough and quite consistent compound scan. It even rang a bell when it finished to recall its attendants.... This machine was in use from 1959 to 1967, working safely and surprisingly reliably, considering its complexity, and with it Donald and his colleagues amassed a very substantial bank of clinical data."[3]

References: 1. McNay MB, Fleming JEE. Fifty Years of Obstetric Ultrasound 1957–1997: From A-Scope to Three Dimensions. *Ultrasound in Medicine and Biology.* 1999; 25(1):7. 2. Ibid. 3. Brown TG. Presentation at the Symposium on the History of Medical Ultrasound. Washington, D.C., 1988. Copy in American Institute of Ultrasound in Medicine archives. Cited in ibid., 10.

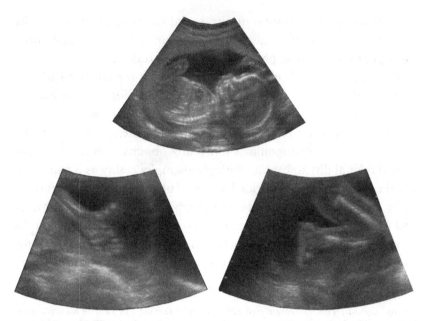

Figure 23. The profile, hand, and leg/foot of a five-month-old fetus taken by ultrasound scanning, 2008.

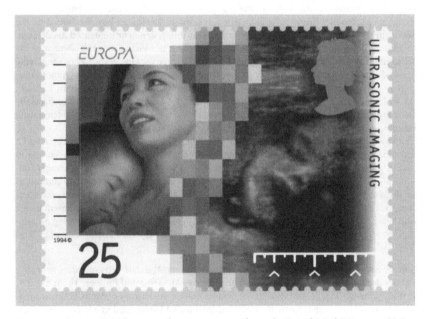

Figure 24. A 1994 British twenty-five-pence stamp from the Royal Mail Discovery Series, titled "Ultrasound Imaging." Stamp designs © Royal Mail Group Ltd. Reproduced by kind permission of Royal Mail Group Ltd. All rights reserved.

from the constraints of objectivity, the photographic and, by extension, the ultrasonic image becomes malleable. The image invites viewers to enter it, to see their social, emotional, and theoretical beliefs expressed in and through it. It is because of this feature that the ultrasound image can be not only a scientific statement but also a cultural artifact laden with personal meanings.

A major concern about ultrasound's social and psychological effects in monitoring pregnancy, expressed in public literature on birthing, stems from its conceptual separation of mother and fetus. It is perceived by some commentators as dividing them into two patients instead of maintaining their relation as a unified pair, and as diminishing the significance of the physical changes and feelings experienced by mothers during pregnancy in favor of its technological depiction through images – a process some women view as objectifying and depersonalizing. What is more, rather than the baby's existence communicated to society through the interpretive experience of the mother who carries it, technology is seen to assume this role: "Picture the diagnostic scene now," writes Rothman,

the woman on the table with the ultrasound scanner to her belly, and on the other side of the technician or doctor, the fetus on the screen. The doctor sits between the mother and the fetus. He turns *away* from the mother to examine her baby. Even the heartbeat is heard over a speaker removed from the mother's body. The technology that makes the baby/fetus more "visible" renders the woman *invisible*. The process works on the woman herself. We now hear women talking about how they felt they "bonded" with their baby when they saw it on the screen. The direct relationship to the baby within them, the fetus as part of their bodies, is superseded by the relationship with the fetus on the screen. The television image becomes more real than the fetus within; it is that image to which they "bond"; it is that image they hold in their minds as they feel their babies move.[16]

The imagery of individualizing and separation of the fetus from the mother had been carried into popular culture in 1968 by the filmmaker Stanley Kubrick, in his legendary work *2001: A Space Odyssey*. The fetus received an astronautlike depiction in the film. It was, as Petchesky wrote: "'a baby man,' an autonomous, atomized space hero.... The image has not supplanted the one of the foetus as a tiny, helpless, suffering creature but rather merged with it."[17] A pregnant woman reflected on such identity issues when seeing her baby on the ultrasound screen: "It was very strange to see the kid and what it was doing. Because the midwife told that it was standing there and covering its eyes with its hands, and waving its hands and . . . almost as if to say something. . . . I know it's happening inside of me, but it was strange anyway [laughs]. Because it looks more like it's happening *out*side."[18] These images portray an independent being in perpetual motion, no longer developing in secret but in stages made public to an audience – medical and familial.

Thus for some women, technologies such as ultrasound raised dilemmas cogently portrayed in feminist literature and summarized by Saetman: "as the fetus gains visibility, the pregnant woman loses visibility and/or autonomy – that her own health, and knowledge, and interests, etc., will be increasingly ignored and her behavior increasingly controlled. There has also been concern that women themselves would lose confidence in their own bodies and their knowledge of their bodies, deferring to physicians to tell them such things as when they got pregnant and how they are faring. . . . In short, there have been numerous and varied concerns for the effects that implementation of [reproductive technologies] might have on women's health, autonomy, and integrity."[19]

The need of a means for health providers and consumers to reconcile the divergent views they hold about the therapies of medicine is exemplified by the problems their different readings of messages broadcast by ultrasound imaging can create. And there is no better means to address this and other significant issues of care than the medium of dialogue. Through it, the views of participants about each other's needs and goals can be aired, and the knowledge they have about the matters that bring them together merged. But in today's medicine, there is a diminished interest in such exchange. "Nobody is talking to patients," observed an American physician in 2008, who pointed to a "broken" health system as the cause.[20] However, the system is guided by and broadly reflects medicine's technological focus and anatomical thinking, the more basic sources of the problem. So, in the face of the doctor's lack of incentive to talk, consumers and patients have turned elsewhere for health dialogue – to one another. This trend, as we have shown, has been demonstrated in the past half century by the rise of self-help groups, social collectives such as those that developed in the women's health movement, and health-related online support communities.

While dialogue in the medical relationship has been problematic, there has been increasing outreach to consumers by society and medicine to assist health professionals in dealing with medical issues having complicated ethical and social dimensions. Such outreach is exemplified by the public committee convened in Seattle in the 1960s to allocate scarce kidney-dialysis machines; the addition of consumer representatives to hospital ethics committees, which have proliferated since the mid-1970s in response to ethical controversies such as the one over keeping Karen Ann Quinlan on a respirator; and the public forums and advisory councils with large citizen representation created in the 1980s and 1990s to reshape health-care provision in Oregon – all events we have previously considered. That a public grown increasingly medically literate is gaining a voice in medical and social decision-making forums betokens a rising tide moving American society toward a more consumer-responsive health system. But to sustain this momentum, the public must stay informed about health care, be ready to assert health views and rights, and maintain a voice in social and medical institutions affecting health-care provision. These efforts deserve the support of physicians, who should recognize that their view of health and illness can be only partial and requires the perspective of the public they care for to complete. Doctor and patient need each other equally; without their collaboration, the promise of medicine is dimmed. But with them acting together, the prospects for medicine are brilliant.

The issues raised in this chapter call for three basic steps to harmonize the technological with the social and humanistic spheres of medicine. The first should be to evaluate the adequacy of the current theoretical basis of medicine. We have explored this matter earlier (see Chapter 7) and shown the advantages of an adaptive concept, which views health and disease as outcomes of interactions individuals have with environments encircling their lives – mainly the outer physical and social worlds and the inner personal and mental one. Accommodative responses to the challenges of these environments are synonymous with wellness, just as unaccommodative ones are with illness. The adaptive perspective was a basic component of Hippocratic medicine, and in the last half of the twentieth century it has been explored most prominently by a microbiologist and professor at the Rockefeller Institute, René Dubos, in books such as *Man Adapting*. Dubos viewed human beings not merely as reacting to the environments of life as did other biological organisms but as consciously responding to them as an expression of human will and strivings. Adaptation thereby had physiological and psychological components. "Human life is thus," wrote Dubos, "the outcome of the interplay between three separate classes of determinants, namely: the lasting and universal characteristics of man's nature, which are inscribed in his flesh and bone; the ephemeral conditions which man encounters at a given moment; and last but not least, man's ability to choose between alternatives and to decide upon a course of action. Ideally, the goal of medicine has always been to help man function successfully in his environment – whether he is hunting the mammoth, toiling for his daily bread, or attempting to reach the moon."[21] Accordingly, an adaptive perspective resists inclinations to view a person's health condition narrowly. It requires synthetic thinking that connects multiple sources of wellness and illness, and the different sorts of facts and truths that can be gathered about them. Anatomical interests and findings can be incorporated into this approach but cannot dominate it. Without an ethos of practice influenced by such a perspective, medicine will remain focused on and largely confined by the vistas displayed through its technology.

The interactive nature of the adaptive concept heightens the significance of a second step needed to master the technology and widen the vision of medicine – establishing strong medical relationships. To understand the living environments and the adaptive capabilities and responses of people, and to use more tellingly the medical insights of informed modern consumers and patients, relationship and the dialogue sustaining it are essential. They generate evidence and resolve problems that technological interventions cannot. Only when the theory explaining health and illness requires relationships and dialogue to thrive will learning the essence of who we are and what we need as patients become a prominent and constant feature of medical encounters.

A third step necessary to encourage the measured use of technology is cogent social policies. Up to now, they have been the most prominent means applied to this effort. Examples are giving fixed payments to treat particular medical problems, regardless of how many technological and other interventions are made, in an effort to limit unnecessary therapies;

and assessing the effectiveness of technologies in terms of their cost, benefits, and burdens compared to alternative treatments, in an attempt to determine the best therapy for given conditions. While essential, as the main agents used to guide technology, social policies have been ineffective. This is because without alternative ways to conceptualize illness that provide nontechnological paths to understand and treat patients, physicians will resist placing limits on what they view as their first and most dependable option – technological measures. How can they do otherwise? To succeed in the goal of rationalizing the use of technology, policy initiatives require a new foundation of relational and conceptual supports. This structure should rise under the banner of a different kind of CPR for medicine: one that joins concepts, policies, and relationships to effectively govern its empire of machines.

NOTES

CHAPTER 1. REVEALING THE BODY'S WHISPERS: HOW THE
STETHOSCOPE TRANSFORMED MEDICINE

1. Hippocrates. Epidemics I. In WHS Jones (ed.). *Hippocrates*, Cambridge, Mass.: Harvard University Press; 1962, 1:187–91.
2. Poynter FNL, Bishop WJ. *A Seventeenth-Century Country Doctor and His Patients: John Symcotts, 1592?–1662*. Streatley: Bedfordshire Historical Record Society; 1951, 31:14.
3. Cullen W. *A Methodical System of Nosology*. Eldad Lewis (trans.). Stockbridge, Mass.: Cornelius Sturtevant; 1808, xxv.
4. Monro A. *The Morbid Anatomy of the Human Gullet, Stomach, and Intestines*. Edinburgh: Archibald Constable and Company; 1811, xxi.
5. O'Malley CD. *Andreas Vesalius of Brussels: 1514–1564*. Berkeley: University of California Press; 1965.
6. Morgagni JB. *The Seats and Causes of Diseases Investigated by Anatomy*. Benjamin Alexander (trans.), with a preface, introduction, and a new translation of five letters by Paul Klemperer. New York: Macmillan, Hafner Publishing; 1960. In this translation, Morgagni's first name was anglicized from Giovanni to John.
7. Laennec RTH. *A Treatise on the Diseases of the Chest*. John Forbes (trans.), 1821 ed. New York: Hafner Publishing; 1962, 285.
8. Ibid., 298.
9. Ibid., 303–4.
10. Ibid., xvii.
11. Magendie F. On Abnormal Sounds in Different Parts of the Human Body. *Boston Medical and Surgical Journal*. 1835; 12:183.
12. Elliotson JE. *The Principles and Practice of Medicine: Founded on the Most Extensive Experience in Public Hospitals and Private Practice, and Developed in a Course of Lectures*. London: Joseph Butler; 1839, xiii.
13. Grant K (ed.). *Memoir of the Late James Hope; by Mrs. Hope...*, 4th ed. London: J. Hatchard & Son; 1848, 75–6.
14. Holmes OW. *Library of Practical Medicine*. Boylston Prize Dissertations for 1836. Boston: Perkins and Marvin; 1836, 7:222.

15. Hughes HM. Illustrations of the Alleged Fallacies of Auscultation, &c. *London Medical Gazette.* 1842–3; 32:418.
16. Review of Stokes' Introduction to the Use of the Stethoscope ... *Lancet.* 1826; 9:472.
17. Latham PM. *Lectures on Subjects Connected with Clinical Medicine.* London: Longman, Bees, Orme, Brown, Green & Longman; 1836, vi.
18. Bell LV. *Library of Practical Medicine.* Boylston Prize Dissertations for 1836. Boston: Perkins and Marvin; 1836, 7:49.
19. Martin R (ed.). *The Collected Works of P.M. Latham.* London: New Sydenham Society; 1876, 1:49.
20. Holmes OW. The Stethoscope Song: A Professional Ballad. In *Poems.* Boston: Tickner, Reed, & Fields; 1850, 272–7. The stopper referred to in the first stanza of the ballad is a piece of wood that could be inserted into (and firmly fit) the flared opening at the patient's end of the stethoscope to hear heart sounds better and to detect lung disorders revealed by changes in the character of the voice as it was transmitted through the chest when the patient spoke. The stopper was a component of Laennec's original stethoscope and described in his 1819 treatise on auscultation. By the mid-nineteenth century, when Holmes wrote this parody, many versions of the stethoscope had appeared. Most were smaller and lighter than Laennec's instrument, and although variously designed and having additions such as the ivory cap mentioned in the parody, they retained its basic tubular form and wooden composition. Stethoscopes made of single lengths of flexible tubing also were developed at this time. They allowed doctors to examine the body with fewer changes in posture required of patients. Such stethoscopes, both the newer wooden and the flexible types, gradually replaced Laennec's model in practice.
21. *Blackwood's Edinburgh Magazine.* March 1847; 61:361.
22. One of the New School. Letter to the Editor, *London Medical Gazette.* 1828; 2:408–9.
23. Review of Duncan's Empyema and Pneumo-Thorax. *Medico-Chirurgical Review.* 1828; 8:131–2.
24. Reply to Drs. Graves' and Stokes' Remarks on Dr. Hope, in Reference to Auscultation. *London Medical Gazette.* 1838–9; 1:129–30.

CHAPTER 2. ENIGMATIC PICTURES: HOW PATIENTS
AND DOCTORS ENCOUNTERED THE X-RAY

1. Vesalius A. *De humani corporis fabrica septre libra.* Basel; 1543.
2. Hooke R. *Micrographia; Or, Some Physiological Descriptions of Minute Bodies Made by Magnifying Glasses with Observations and Inquiries Thereupon.* London: Jo. Marlyn and Ja. Allestry; 1665.
3. Lane JE. Bonomo's Letter to Redi: An Important Document in the History of Scabies. *Archives of Dermatology and Syphilology.* 1928; 18:22–4.
4. Schierbeek A. *Measuring the Invisible World: The Life and Works of Antoni van Leeuwenhoek. FRS.* London: Abelard – Schuman; 1959, 72.
5. Fox DM, Lawrence C. *Photographing Medicine: Images and Power in Britain and America since 1840.* New York: Greenwood Press; 1988.

6. Koch R. Investigations on Tuberculosis. *British Medical Journal.* 1882; 1:707; Koch R. Investigation of Pathogenic Organisms. In WW Cheyne (ed.), *Recent Essays by Various Authors on Bacteria in Relation to Disease.* London: New Sydenham Society; 1886, 26–32.
7. Sontag S. *On Photography.* New York: Doubleday; 1977; Berger J. Uses of Photography. In G. Dryer (ed.), *John Berger: Selected Essays.* New York: Pantheon Books; 2001, 279–82; Gernsheim H, Gernsheim A. *A Concise History of Photography.* London: Thames & Hudson; 1971, 48.
8. Glasser O. *Dr. W. C. Roentgen.* Springfield, Ill.: Charles C. Thomas; 1958.
9. Röntgen W. On a New Kind of Rays, a Preliminary Communication. In O. Glasser, op. cit., 41–52.
10. Ibid., 39.
11. Ibid., 57, 82, 90.
12. Her Latest Photograph. *New York Times,* May 29, 1898, 14.
13. Brecher R, Brecher E. *The Rays: A History of Radiology in the United States and Canada.* Baltimore: Williams and Wilkins; 1969, 33.
14. Ibid., 65.
15. Ibid., 61.
16. Ibid., 63, 59–60.
17. Ibid., 86.
18. Duffin J, Hayter CRR. Baring the Sole: The Rise and Fall of the Shoe-Fitting Fluoroscope. *Isis.* 2000; 91, 260–82.
19. Instruments Collection. Francis A. Countway Library of Medicine, Boston.
20. Stethoscope Versus X-rays. *British Medical Journal.* 1945; 2:856.
21. Brecher, op. cit., 217.
22. Jauhar S. Restoring the Physical to the Exam. *New York Times.* January 29, 2002, D6.
23. Pearson K. *The Grammar of Science.* London: Adam and Charles Black; 1900.
24. Berger, op. cit., 287.
25. Berkelo CC et al. Tuberculosis Case Findings. *JAMA.* 1947; 133, 354–65.
26. Garland LH. On the Scientific Evaluation of Diagnostic Procedures. *Radiology.* 1949; 52:312.
27. Reiser SJ. *Medicine and the Reign of Technology.* New York: Cambridge University Press; 1978, 174–95.

CHAPTER 3. LIFESAVING BUT UNAFFORDABLE: THE IMPROBABLE
JOURNEY OF THE ARTIFICIAL KIDNEY

1. Van Noordwijk J. *Dialysing for Life: The Development of the Artificial Kidney.* Dordrecht, The Netherlands: Kluwer Academic Publishers; 2001, 5.
2. Kolff WJ. First Clinical Experience with the Artificial Kidney. *Annals of Internal Medicine.* 1965; 62:608.
3. Graham T. Osmotic Force. *Philosophical Transactions Royal Society of London.* 1854; 144:177–228.
4. McBridge P. The Development of Hemodialysis and Peritoneal Dialysis. In Nissenson AR, Fine RM, Gentile DE. *Clinical Dialysis,* 3rd ed. Norwalk, Conn.: Appelton & Longe; 1995, 3.

5. Abel J, Rountree L, Turner B. On the Removal of Diffusible Substances from the Circulating Blood of Living Animals by Dialysis. *Journal of Pharmacological Experimental Therapy.* 1914; 5:275–316.
6. McBridge, op. cit., 4–5.
7. Van Noordwijk, op. cit., 8–11.
8. Kolff, op. cit., 608.
9. Ibid., 609.
10. Van Noordwijk, op. cit., 1, 3.
11. Kolff, op. cit., 617.
12. Ibid.
13. Van Noordwijk, op. cit., 23–6, 42–3.
14. Kolff, op. cit., 615.
15. Teschan P et al. Prophylactic Hemodialysis in the Treatment of Acute Renal Failure. *Annals of Internal Medicine.* 1960; 53.
16. Altman LH. Dr. Belding H. Scribner, Medical Pioneer, Is Dead at 82. *New York Times,* June 22, 2003, 25.
17. Kolff WJ. *Artificial Organs.* New York: John Wiley & Sons; 1976, 132. See also Sanders I, Dukeminier J. Medical Advance and Legal Lag: Hemodialysis and Kidney Transplantation. *UCLA Law Review.* 1968; 15:361.
18. The average cost per patient of dialysis at the Seattle Center of $10,000 was maintained in the center's first years, which was lower than was possible in most other places because of government grants and other contributions to the center. In 1966 in Los Angeles, for example, dialysis at Wadsworth Veterans Administration Hospital was as much as $28,000 a year. The high cost of dialysis for chronic kidney disease was due to three main factors: its space requirements in hospitals, the price of the kidney machine, and the need for personnel who were specially trained. Sanders and Dukeminier, op. cit., 362.
19. Haviland JW. Experiences in Establishing a Community Artificial Kidney Center. *Transactions of the American Clinical and Climatological Association.* 1966; 77:125–36.
20. Ibid., 132, table 4.
21. Alexander S. They Decide Who Lives, Who Dies. *Life,* Nov. 2, 1962, 102–10, 115–18, 123–5.
22. Ibid., 110.
23. Ibid., 115–18, 123.
24. Ibid., 125.
25. Kolff, op. cit., First, 618.
26. Sanders and Dukeminier, op. cit., 378.
27. Ibid., 366–7.
28. Sanders and Dukeminier, op. cit., 366.
29. Robbins Jhan, Robbins June. The Rest Are Simply Left to Die. *Redbook,* Nov. 1967, 132.
30. Ibid., 134.
31. Gottschalk CW. Commentary. In Hanna KE (ed.) *Biomedical Politics.* Washington, D.C.: National Academy Press; 1991, 210.
32. Rettig RA. Origins of the Medicare Kidney Disease Entitlement: The Social Security Amendments of 1972. In Hanna, op. cit., 182.

33. Ibid., 187.
34. Ibid., 189.
35. Ibid., 204.
36. The Robert Wood Johnson Foundation. *High and Rising Health Care Costs: Demystifying U.S. Health Care Spending.* Research Synthesis Report No. 16. Princeton, NJ; 2008, 3–4, 11–17.

CHAPTER 4. PROMISING RESCUE, PREVENTING RELEASE: THE DOUBLE EDGE OF THE ARTIFICIAL RESPIRATOR

1. Eross B, Pouner D, Grenvik A. Historical Survey of Mechanical Ventilation. *International Anesthesiology Clinics.* 1980; 18:1–10.
2. Hilberman M. The Evolution of Intensive Care Units. *Critical Care Medicine.* 1975; 3:159–65.
3. Woollam CHM. The Development of Apparatus for Intermittent Negative Pressure Respiration. *Anaesthesia.* 1976; 31:537–47.
4. With the invention of effective anesthetics (ether in 1846 and chloroform in 1847) and the control of sources of surgical infections (explicated between 1875 and 1880), hospital surgery flourished by the twentieth century (see Chapter 8).
5. Eross, Pouner, and Grenvik, op. cit., 2–3.
6. Drinker P, Shaw LA. The Prolonged Administration of Artificial Respiration. *Journal of the Franklin Institute.* 1932; 213:356–7.
7. Drinker P, McKhann CF. The Use of a New Apparatus for the Prolonged Administration of Artificial Respiration. *JAMA.* 1929; 92:1658–60; Drinker and Shaw, op. cit., 365–6.
8. Drinker and McKhann, op. cit., 1658.
9. Paul J. *History of Poliomyelitis.* New Haven, Conn.: Yale University Press; 1971, 327.
10. Maxwell JH. The Iron Lung: Halfway Technology or Necessary Step? *Milbank Quarterly.* 1986; 64:3–29.
11. Ibid., 10–11. Wilson JL. The Use of the Respirator. *JAMA.* 1941; 17:278–9.
12. Paul, op. cit., 330–1.
13. Ibid., 311–12.
14. Maxwell, op. cit., 13–15.
15. Anderson EW, Ibsen B. The Anaesthetic Management of Patients with Poliomyelitis and Respiratory Paralysis. *British Medical Journal.* 1954; 1:786–8.
16. Lassen HCA. A Preliminary Report on the 1952 Epidemic of Poliomyelitis in Copenhagen. *Lancet.* 1953; 1:37–41.
17. Hilberman, op. cit., 161.
18. Maxwell, op. cit., 18.
19. Pope Pius XII. The Prolongation of Life. *The Pope Speaks.* 1958; 4:393–8.
20. Panicola M. Catholic Teaching on Prolonging Life: Setting the Record Straight. *Hastings Center Report.* 2001; 31(6):14–25.
21. Sanders D, Dukeminier J. Medical Advance and Legal Lag: Hemodialysis and Kidney Transplantation. *UCLA Law Review.* 1968; 15:408.
22. Ibid., 388.

23. Ibid., 394.
24. Ibid., 408.
25. Committee of the Harvard Medical School. A Definition of Irreversible Coma: Report of the Ad Hoc Committee of the Harvard Medical School to Examine the Definition of Brain Death. *JAMA*. 1968; 205:337–40.
26. Supreme Court of New Jersey, 70 N.J. 10, 355A, 2d647 (1976).
27. Teel K. The Physician's Dilemma: A Doctor's View: What the Law Should Be. *Baylor Law Review*. 1975; 27:6, 8–9.
28. Hippocrates. The Art. In Jones WHS (trans.), *Hippocrates*. Cambridge, Mass.: Harvard University Press; 1962, 1:317, 319.
29. California Natural Death Act of 1976. In Reiser SJ, Dyck AJ, Curran WJ (eds.), *Ethics in Medicine: Historical Perspectives and Contemporary Concerns*. Cambridge, Mass.: MIT Press; 1977, 665–7.
30. Gotbaum R. A Beautiful Death. *Proto: Massachusetts General Hospital Dispatches from the Frontiers of Medicine*. Fall 2005. An interview with Dr. Ned Cassem, a psychiatrist and Jesuit priest who established the Optimum Care Committee at MGH in 1973 to deal with end-of-life issues and called it the first ethics consultation committee formed in North America. The committee continues to function under this name.
31. Fine RL, Mayo TW. Resolution of Futility by Due Process: Early Experience with the Texas Advance Directives Act. *Annals of Internal Medicine*. 2003; 138:743–7.
32. Helft PR, Siegler M, Lantos J. The Rise and Fall of the Futility Movement. *New England Journal of Medicine*. 2000; 343:293–6.

CHAPTER 5. THE QUEST TO UNIFY HEALTH CARE THROUGH
THE PATIENT RECORD

1. Jackson J. Appendix. In Louis PCA, *Researches on the Effects of Bloodletting*, Putnam CG (trans.). Boston: Hilliard, Gray, and Company; 1836, 100–2.
2. Reiser SJ. Creating Form out of Mass: The Development of the Medical Record. In Mendelsohn E (ed.), *Transformation and the Sciences: Essays in Honor of I. Bernard Cohen*. (Cambridge: Cambridge University Press); 1984, 303–16.
3. Marey E-J. The Graphic Method on the Experimental Sciences and Its Special Application in Medicine. *British Medical Journal*; 1876, 1:1–3, 63–6.
4. Chambers TK. Drill for Auscultation. *The Lancet*; 1861, 1:334.
5. Nightingale F. *Notes on Hospitals*. London: Longman Green; 1863, 175–6.
6. Clapesattle H. *The Doctors Mayo*. Minneapolis: University of Minnesota Press; 1941, 385.
7. Cannon WB. The Case Method Applied to Medicine. *Boston Medical and Surgical Journal*; 1900, 142:32.
8. Washburn FA. *The Massachusetts General Hospital: Its Development, 1900–1935*. Boston: Houghton Mifflin; 1939, 115–16.
9. Painter FM. Extending the Influence of a Hospital. *The Modern Hospital*; 1918, 2:356.
10. Reiser SJ. The Clinical Record in Medicine. Part I: Learning from Cases. *Annals of Internal Medicine*. 1991; 114(10):907.

11. Neuhauser D. Ernest Amory Codman and the End Results of Medical Care. In Introduction to Codman EA, *A Study in Hospital Efficiency*, 1917. Oakbrook Terrace, Ill.: Joint Commission on Accreditation of Healthcare Organizations; 1996, 11–12.
12. Codman EA. Case-Records and Their Value. *Bulletin of the American College of Surgeons*; 1917, 3:24–7.
13. Bowman JG. Introduction to Case Records and Their Use. *Bulletin of the American College of Surgeons*; 1919, 4:2–3.
14. Codman EA, op. cit., 112.
15. Hornsby J. The Hospital Problem of Today – What Is It? *Bulletin of the American College of Surgeons*; 1917, 3:7.
16. Hospital Standardization Series: General Hospitals of 100 or More Beds. *Bulletin of the American College of Surgeons*; 1919, 4–5.
17. Peebles A. *A Survey of Medical Facilities of Shelby County, Indiana*. Washington, D.C.: Committee on the Costs of Medical Care, 1919.
18. Peterson O et al. *An Analytic Study of North Carolina General Practice, 1953–1954*. Evanston, Ill.: Association of American Medical Colleges; 1956, 24.
19. Evans JL. Access to Patients' Records. *Bulletin of the American College of Surgeons*; 1924, 8:55.
20. Long JW. Case Records in Hospitals. *Bulletin of the American College of Surgeons*; 1924, 8:65.
21. Auchincloss H. Unit History System. In *Methods and Problems of Medical Education*, 4th ser. New York: Rockefeller Foundation; 1926.
22. Corscaden JH. Follow-up System. In ibid., 27–32.
23. Pearl R. Modern Methods in Handling Hospital Statistics. *Johns Hopkins Bulletin*; 1921, 8:186.
24. Ibid., 187–8.
25. Reiser SJ. *Medicine and the Reign of Technology*. New York: Cambridge University Press; 1978, 208–10.
26. Crebink GA, Hurst L. *Computer Projects in Health Care*. Ann Arbor, Mich.: Health Administration Press; 1975, 5–6.
27. Feinstein A. *Clinical Judgment*. Baltimore: Williams and Wilkens; 1967.
28. Weed LL. *Medical Records, Medical Education, and Patient Care*. Cleveland, Ohio: Press of Case Western Reserve University; 1971, 247–50.
29. Fisher PJ, Statmarin WC, Lundsgaarde HP, et al. User Reaction to PROMIS: Issues Related to Acceptability of Medical Innovations. In O' Neill JT (ed.), *Proceedings: Fourth Annual Symposium on Computer Applications in Medical Care*. New York: Institute of Electrical and Electronic Engineers, 1980, 1722–30.
30. Reiser, op. cit., Creating, 303–16.
31. Mauliner C, Ramsey GA, Kempwood, RC. *Case Records. Bulletin of the American College of Surgeons*. 1923; 7:23.
32. Grossman JH. Physicians as Managers in Hospitals. Paper prepared for delivery at King's Fund Centre for Health Services Development; 1989, 4.
33. Dick RS, Steen EB (eds.). *The Computer-Based Patient Record: An Essential Technology for Health Care*. Washington, D.C.: National Academy Press; 1991, 2–3.

34. Kohn LT, Corrigan JM, Donaldson MS (eds.). *To Err Is Human: Building Safer Health Systems*. Washington, D.C.: National Academy Press; 2000, 178.
35. Sidorow J. It Ain't Necessarily So: The Electronic Health Record and the Unlikely Prospect of Reducing Healthcare Costs. *Health Affairs* 2006; 25 (4): 1079–85. See also Lohr S. Most Doctors Aren't Using Electronic Health Records. *New York Times*. June 19, 2008, C3. Veterans Affairs (VA) medical centers have been significant users of electronic health records and exemplars of their possibilities. For a discussion of the benefits and problems their use has produced in the VA system see: Evans DC, Nichol PW, Perlon JA. Effect of the Implementation of an Enterprise-wide Electronic Health Record on Productivity in the Veterans Health Administration. *Health Economics Policy and Law*. 2006; 42:163–4; Kuehn BM. IT Vulnerabilities Highlighted by Errors, Malfunctions at Veterans' Medical Centers. *JAMA*. 2009; 301:919–20. One of the first clinical studies to test the claims of advocates and critics of the electronic health record by measuring the influence of clinical information technologies on inpatient mortality, complications, the cost of care and the length of hospital stays, and which found a positive influence on these outcomes of care is: Amarasingham R, Plantinga L, Diener-West M, et al. Clinical Information Technologies and Inpatient Outcomes: A Multiple Hospital Study. *Archives of Internal Medicine*. 2009; 169: 108–14.
36. Leavitt M. Connecting the Medical Dots. *Washington Post*, Dec. 22, 2008, A21. For an examination of the influence of the economic stimulus bill on electronic medical records see: Conference Report on H.R. 1, American Recovery and Reinvestment Act, 2009. *Congressional Record*: Feb. 12, 2009 (House), H1337–H1350; Yourish K, Stanton L. Breakdown of the Final Bill. *Washington Post*, Feb. 14, 2009, A11; Huslin A. Online Health Data in Remission. *Washington Post*, Feb. 16, 2009, D1, 03. A critical commentary on the bill's endorsement of electronic medical records is, Saumerai SB and Majumdar SR. Bad Bet on Medical Records. *Washington Post*. March 17, 2009, A15.
37. Hartzband P, Groopman J. Off the Record – Avoiding the Pitfalls of Going Electronic. *New England Journal of Medicine*. 2008; 358(16):1656–8. See also Armstrong-Cobed A. The Computer Will See You Now. *New York Times*, March 6, 2009, A-27.
38. Rampell C. Your Health Data, Plugged into the Web. *Washington Post*. Oct. 5, 2007, D1–D2. Lawton C, Worthen B. Google to Offer Health Records on the Web. *Wall Street Journal*, Feb. 28, 2008, D1, D4.
39. Steinbrook R. Personally Controlled Online Health Data – The Next Big Thing in Medical Care? *New England Journal of Medicine*. 2008; 358(16):1653–6. See also Halamka JD, Kennth DM, Tang PC. Early Experiences with Personal Health Records. *Journal of the American Medical Informatics Association*. 2008; 15:1–7.
40. Hippocrates. The Oath. In WHS Jones (ed.), *Hippocrates*. Cambridge, Mass.: Harvard University Press; 1962, 164–5.
41. Pear R. Privacy Issue Complicates Push to Link Medical Data. *New York Times*, Jan. 11, 2009, 11, 14. See also U.S. Department of Health and Human Services. Protecting the Privacy of Patients' Health Information (Fact Sheet). Available at http://www.hhs.gov/news/facts/privacy/html.

42. Reiser SJ. Malpractice, Patient Safety, and the Ethical and Scientific Foundations of Medicine. In Huber PW, Litan RE (eds.), *The Liability Maze: The Impact of Liability Law on Safety and Innovation*. Washington, D.C.: Brookings Institution; 1990, 227–50.

43. Institutions have rights over the record as a physical object, but the patients about whom the record is written own its contents.

CHAPTER 6. PUTTING TECHNOLOGIES ON TRIAL: FROM
BLOODLETTING TO ANTIBIOTICS TO THE OREGON INITIATIVE

1. Brain P. *Galen on Bloodletting*. Cambridge: Cambridge University Press; 1986, 1–14.

2. Reiss O. *Medicine in Colonial America*. Lanham, Md.: University Press of America; 2000, 167–79, 434.

3. Louis PCA. *Researches on the Effects of Bloodletting in Some Inflammatory Diseases*. Putnam CG (trans.). Boston: Hilliard, Gray and Co.; 1836. Reprint; Birmingham, Ala.: Classics of Medicine Library; 1986, v.

4. Ibid., 1.

5. Ibid., 83–4.

6. Ibid., 66.

7. Ibid., 68–9.

8. Matthews JR. *Quantification and the Quest for Medical Certainty*. Princeton, N.J.: Princeton University Press; 30–2.

9. Feinberg SE. Randomization and Social Affairs: The 1970 Draft Lottery. *Science*. 1971; 171:255–61.

10. Chalmers I. Comparing Like with Like: Some Historical Milestones in the Evolution of Methods to Create Unbiased Comparison Groups in Therapeutic Situations. *International Journal of Epidemiology*. 2001; 30: 1157.

11. Ibid., 1158–9.

12. Clinical Trials: A Cornerstone of Biomedical Research and Innovation. *Pfizer Journal*. 2002; 3(1):8.

13. Frazier HS, Mosteller F. *Medicine Worth Paying For: Assessing Medical Innovations*. Cambridge, Mass.: Harvard University Press; 1995, 11.

14. Chalmers, op. cit., 1160.

15. Ibid., 1161.

16. Kaptchuk TI. Intentional Ignorance: A History of Blind Assessment and Placebo Controls in Medicine. *Bulletin of the History of Medicine*. 1998; 72:395–7.

17. Ibid., 420–1.

18. Ibid., 427–8.

19. Matthews, op. cit., 127–9.

20. Hill AB. The Aim of the Statistical Method. *The Lancet*. 1937; 1:43.

21. The Controlled Therapeutic Trial. Editorial in *British Medical Journal*. 1948; 2:791–2.

22. Hill AB. Suspended Judgement: Memories of the British Streptomycin Trial in Tuberculosis: The First Randomized Clinical Trial. *Controlled Clinical Trials*. 1990; 11:77.

23. Yoshioka A. Use of Randomization in the Medical Research Council's Clinical Trial of Streptomycin in Pulmonary Tuberculosis in the 1940s. *British Medical Journal*. 1998; 317:1220.

24. Matthews, op. cit., 129.

25. Yoshioka, op. cit., 1220.

26. Hill, op. cit., Suspended, 78.

27. Medical Research Council. Streptomycin Treatment of Pulmonary Tuberculosis. *British Medical Journal*. 1948; 2:769–70.

28. Chalmers, op. cit., 1162.

29. Doll R. Controlled Trials: The 1948 Watershed. *British Medical Journal*. 1998; 317:1217–20.

30. Hill AB. Medical Ethics and Controlled Trials. *British Medical Journal*. 1963; 1:1043.

31. Medical Research Council, op. cit., 780.

32. Dickersin K, Rennie O. Registering Clinical Trials. *JAMA*. 2003; 290:516.

33. Frazier and Mosteller, op. cit., 24–5, 246–7.

34. Dickersin and Rennie, op. cit., 517.

35. Krzyzanowska MK, Pinitilee M, Tannock IF. Factors Associated with Failure to Publish Large Randomized Trials Presented at an Oncology Meeting. *JAMA*. 2003; 290:495–501.

36. De Angelis CD, Drazen JM, Frizelle FA, et al. Clinical Trial Registration: A Statement from the International Committee of Medical Journal Editors. *JAMA*. 2004; 292:1363–4.

37. De Angelis CD, Drazen JM, Frizelle FA, et al. Is This Clinical Trial Fully Registered? A Statement From the International Committee of Medical Journal Editors. *JAMA*. 2005; 293:2927–9.

38. U.S. Congress, Office of Technology Assessment. *Evaluation of the Oregon Medicaid Proposal (OTA-H-531)*. Washington, D.C.: U.S. Government Printing Office; 1992, 1–3. Thorne JI. The Oregon Plan Approach to Comprehensive and Rational Health Care. In Strosberg MA, Wiener JM, Baker R, Fein IA. *Rationing America's Medical Care: The Oregon Plan and Beyond*. Washington, D.C.: Brookings Institution; 1992, 24–9.

39. Garland MI. Rationing in Public: Oregon's Priority-Setting Methodology. In Strosberg et al., op. cit., 37–8.

40. U.S. Congress, Office of Technology Assessment, op. cit., 40–1. Hadorn DC. The Oregon Priority-Setting Exercise: Quality of Life and Public Policy. In Beauchamp TL, Walters L (eds.), *Contemporary Issues in Bioethics*. Belmont, Calif.: Wadsworth Publishing; 1994, 734.

41. U.S. Congress, Office of Technology Assessment, op. cit., 48.

42. Ibid., 9.

43. Ibid., 50.

44. Kaplan RM. A Quality-of-Life Approach to Health Resource Allocation. In Strosberg et al., op. cit., 75.

45. Veatch RM. The Oregon Experiment: Needless and Real Worries. In ibid., 83.

46. Rosenbaum S. Poor Women, Poor Children, Poor Policy: The Oregon Medical Experiment. In ibid., 91–2.

47. La Puma J. Quality-Adjusted Life-Years: Why Physicians Should Reject Oregon's Plan. In ibid., 125–6.
48. Tartaglia AP. Is Talk of Rationing Premature? In ibid., 144–50.
49. Daniels N. Justice and Health Care Rationing: Lessons from Oregon. In ibid., 194.
50. Baker R. The Inevitability of Health Care Rationing: A Case Study of Rationing in the British National Health Service. In ibid., 225.
51. Wyden RL. Why I Support the Oregon Plan. In ibid., 115.
52. U.S. Congress, Office of Technology Assessment, op. cit., 20–1.
53. Callahan D. Ethics and Priority Setting in Oregon. In Beauchamp and Walters, op. cit., 750–1.

CHAPTER 7. AMID THE TECHNOLOGICAL TRIUMPHS OF DISEASE
PREVENTION – WHERE IS HEALTH?

1. Toby JA. The Health Examination Movement. *The Nation's Health*. 1923; 5(9):610–11, 648–9.
2. Hippocrates. Airs, Waters, Places. In Adams F (trans.), *The Genuine Works of Hippocrates*. London: Sydenham Society; 1849. Reprinted in Classics of Medicine Library. Birmingham, Ala.: 1985; 190–1.
3. Hippocrates. The Physician. In Jones WHF (trans.), *Hippocrates*. Cambridge, Mass.: Harvard University Press; 1962, 2:193.
4. Sydenham T. Medical Observations Concerning the History and Cure of Acute Diseases. In Latham RG (trans.), *The Works of Thomas Sydenham*. London: Sydenham Society; 1848–50, 15.
5. Clendening L. *Behind the Doctor*. Garden City, NY: Garden City Publishing; 1933, 156.
6. Sydenham, op. cit., 19.
7. Morgagni JB. *The Seats and Causes of Diseases Investigated by Anatomy*. Benjamin Alexander (trans.). New York: Macmillan, Hafner Press; 1960, 1:xxx. See also comment in note 6, Chapter 1.
8. Ibid., xxiv.
9. Virchow R. The Influence of Morgagni on Anatomical Thought. *The Lancet*. 1894; 1:846.
10. Koch's Investigations on Tuberculosis. *British Medical Journal*. 1882; 1: 707.
11. Kraut AM. Silent Travelers: Germs, Genes, and the "Immigrant Menace." Baltimore: Johns Hopkins University Press; 1994, 226–7.
12. Reiser SJ. The Emergence of the Concept of Screening for Disease. *Millbank Fund Quarterly*. 1978; 56(4):403–25.
13. Kraut, op. cit., 236, 241.
14. Clark WI. Physical Examination and Medical Supervision of Factory Employees. *Boston Medical and Surgical Journal*. 1917; 176(7):239–44.
15. Reiser, op. cit.
16. Ibid.
17. Toby JA, op. cit.
18. Emerson H. The Protection of Health through Periodic Medical Examinations. *Journal of the Michigan Medical Society*. 1922; 21(9):399–403.

19. Fremont-Smith H. Periodic Examination of Supposedly Well Persons. *New England Journal of Medicine.* 1953; 248(5):170–3.

20. Reiser, op. cit.

21. The Complete Physical Examination. *New England Journal of Medicine.* 1957; 256(17):814–15.

22. Woolf SH. The Accuracy and Effectiveness of Routine Population Screening with Mammography, Prostate-Specific Antigen, and Prenatal Ultrasound: A Review of Published Scientific Evidence. *International Journal of Technology Assessment in Health Care.* 2001; 17(3):276–304.

23. Getting VA. Mass Screening or the Multiphasic Clinic. *Journal of the Michigan Medical Society.* 1951; 50(7):726–9.

24. Thorner RM. Whither Multiphasic Screening? *New England Journal of Medicine.* 1969; 280(19):1037–42.

25. Peckham CS, Dezateux C. Issues Underlying the Evaluation of Screening Programmes. *British Medical Bulletin.* 1998; 54(4):767–78. (This is the introductory essay to an informative issue of the *Bulletin* on screening.)

26. Ibid.

27. Kessler HH. The Determination of Physical Fitness. *JAMA.* 1940; 115(19):1591–5.

28. Rosen G. A History of Public Health. New York: MD Publications; 1958:234–44.

29. World Health Organization. *Basic Documents*, 35th ed. Geneva; 1985.

30. Breslow L. From Disease to Health Promotion. *JAMA.* 1999; 281(11):1030–3. See also Justice B. *A Different Kind of Health: Finding Well-Being Despite Illness.* Houston: Peak Press: 1998.

31. Green LW, Poland BD, Rootman I. The Settings Approach to Health Promotion. In Poland BD, Green LW, Rootman I (eds.), *Settings for Health Promotion: Linking Theory and Practice.* Thousand Oaks, Calif.: Sage Publications; 2000, 16.

32. Topol E, Murray S, Frazer KA. The Genomics Gold Rush. *JAMA.* 2007; 298(2):218–21.

33. Ibid.

34. Smillie WG. Inherent Inadequacies of Multiphasic Screenings. *JAMA.* 1951; 145(16):1254–6.

35. Reiser SJ. Medicine and Public Health: Pursuing a Common Destiny. *JAMA.* 1996; 276(17):1429–30.

36. As a founder and the National Coordinator of the Medicine/Public Health Initiative from 1994 to 1998, the author introduced the idea of creating a common view of health and illness into its agenda. It was specified as one of the initiative's seven goals, but with other pressing objectives to attain, it was never addressed.

CHAPTER 8. THE TECHNOLOGICAL TRANSFORMATION OF BIRTH

1. Smellie W. A Treatise on the Theory and Practice of Midwifery. London: D. Wilson; 1752. Facsimile reprint; Birmingham, Ala.: Classics of Medicine Library; 1990, 264–5.

2. Leavitt JW. "Science" Enters the Birthing Room: Obstetrics in America since the Eighteenth Century. In Ogawa T (ed.), *History of Obstetrics: Proceedings of the 7th International Symposium on the Comparative History of Medicine – East and West.* Osaka, Japan: Tanigauchi Foundation; 1983, 14.

3. Donnison J. *Midwives and Medical Men: A History of the Struggle for the Control of Childbirth.* London: Historical Publications; 1988, 11–22.

4. Laget M. Practices of Midwives and Obstetricians in France during the Eighteenth Century. In Ogawa, op. cit., 57–74.

5. Loudon I. Death in Childbirth: An International Study of Maternal Care and Maternal Mortality, 1800–1950. Oxford, U.K.: Clarendon Press; 1992, 167.

6. Hibbard B. *The Obstetrician's Armamentariun: Historical Obstetric Instruments and Their Inventors.* San Anselmo, Calif.: Norman Publishing; 2000, 9–16. Beatty W. The History of Obstetric Forceps. *Medical Reflections on Obstetrics and Gynecology.* 1976; 1(4):2–3. Cianfrani T. *A Short History of Obstetrics and Gynecology.* Springfield, Ill.: Charles C. Thomas; 1960, 189–204. Findley P. *The Priests of Lucina: The Story of Obstetrics.* Boston: Little, Brown; 1939, 306–23.

7. Beatty, op. cit., 6.

8. Hibbard, op. cit., 13–14.

9. Towler J, Bramall J. *Midwives in History and Society.* London: Croom Helm; 1986, 79.

10. Beatty, op. cit., 5.

11. Gladwell M. In the Air. *New Yorker.* May 12, 2008, 50–60.

12. Wilbanks ER. Development of Obstetrics as a Medical Specialty. *Medical Reflections in Obstetrics and Gynecology.* 1976; 1(2):6.

13. Ramsey M. Property Rights and the Right to Health: The Regulation of Secret Remedies in France, 1789–1815. In Bynum WF, Porter R (eds.), *Medical Fringe and Medical Orthodoxy 1750–1850.* London: Croom Helm, 1987, 79, 100.

14. An early printed reference to the Chamberlen forceps appears in a book by the English surgeon Edmund Chapman, *An Essay on the Improvement of Midwifery*... London: A. Blackwell, 1733. In it, Chapman praises the forceps, urges his colleagues to apply it, and indicates that for at least twenty-five years the instrument had been used by practitioners in the community but rarely discussed publicly (Cianfrani, op. cit., 201). Apparently, the secrecy with which the Chamberlens shrouded the innovation continued in place among its subsequent early users.

15. Radcliffe W. *The Secret Instrument: The Birth of the Midwifery Forceps.* London: William Heinemann; 1947, 56, 61.

16. Loudon ISL. Childbirth. In Bynum WF, Porter R (eds.), *Companion Encyclopedia of the History of Medicine.* London: Routledge; 1993, 1053.

17. Ellis H. *Famous Operations.* Media, Penn.: Harwal Publishing; 1984, 56–7.

18. Pervical T. Medical Ethics. In Reiser SJ, Curran WJ, Dyck AJ (eds.). *Ethics in Medicine: Historical Perspectives and Contemporary Concerns.* Cambridge, Mass.: MIT Press; 1977, 24.

19. Baskett TF. Edinburgh Connections in a Painful World. *Surgeon;* 2005, 3(2):103.

20. Clark RB. Fanny Longfellow and Nathan Keep. *American Society of Anesthesiologists Newsletter.* 1997; 61(9):7–9.
21. Shephard DAE. Analgesia in Labor Becomes Respectable: The Role of John Snow. *American Society of Anesthesiologists Newsletter.* 1997; 6(9):1–13. See also Drife J. The Start of Life: A History of Obstetrics. *Postgraduate Medical Journal* 2002; 78:313.
22. Leavitt JW. *Brought to Bed: Childbearing in America 1750 to 1950.* New York: Oxford University Press; 1986, 121–2.
23. Parsons GP. The British Medical Profession and Contagion Theory: Puerperal Fever as a Case Study, 1830–1860. *Medical History.* 1978; 22:140.
24. Drife, op. cit., 313.
25. Holmes OW. The Contagiousness of Puerperal Fever. *New England Quarterly Journal of Medicine.* 1843; 1:529–30.
26. Carter KC. Semmelweis and His Predecessors. *Medical History.* 1981; 25:57–72.
27. Humphreys D. *Canadian Medical Association Journal.* 2008; 178(2):194.
28. Ellis, op. cit., 67.
29. Drife, op. cit.; Loudon, op. cit., 1058.
30. Leavitt, "Science," op. cit., 34–5.
31. The case records are thoughtfully portrayed and analyzed in Dye NS. Modern Obstetrics and Working Class Women: The New York Midwifery Dispensary, 1890–1920. *Journal of Social History.* 1987; 20:549–64. The institution whose 1890–1913 records are examined in Dye's essay began in 1890 as the Midwife Dispensary. It changed its name to the New York Lying-In Hospital in 1893, when it merged with the Society for the Lying-In of the City of New York.
32. Ibid., 557.
33. Ibid., 558.
34. Ibid., 560.
35. Leavitt, *Brought,* op. cit., 163–4. The term *meddlesome midwifery* found at the beginning of this quotation is a phrase from the nineteenth century, meaning excessive medical interventions made during birth.
36. Loudon I. Obstetrics and the General Practitioner. *British Medical Journal.* 1990; 301:704. Loudon, Childbirth, op. cit., 1061.
37. In 1955, 95 percent of American births occurred in hospitals. This figure has remained basically stable over time, rising to 99 percent by 2005, when about 65 percent of the 1 percent of out-of-hospital births occurred in homes and 27 percent in freestanding birth centers. Leavitt, *Brought,* op. cit., 269. National Center for Health Statistics, Hyattsville, Md. Births: Final Data for 2005.
38. Pincus J. Introduction to Boston Women's Health Book Collective. *Our Bodies, Ourselves: For the New Century.* New York: Simon and Schuster; 1998, 21.
39. Avery B. Preface to ibid., 15.
40. Luce J, Pincus J, with Levine A. Childbirth, in Boston Women's Health Book Collective, op. cit., 466.
41. Ibid., 469.

42. An index of the growth of technological interventions in birth during the past half century in America has been the rising use of the cesarean section operation to deliver babies. It has grown from about one in twenty in 1965 to more than one in four by 2003 and almost one in three by 2006.[1] One source of this increase has been the widening use of the electronic fetal monitor (EFM) to detect fetal distress by recording the fetal heart rate during labor and delivery. Developed by Edward Hon in 1957, and originally intended for use in high-risk pregnancies, its application gradually has become routine. By 2002 about 3.4 million fetuses (or 85 percent of the some 4 million live American births that year) were monitored with the device, and it was the most commonly used obstetric procedure.[2] But gradually its dependability has been questioned, leading the American College of Obstetrics and Gynecology to state in 2002: "the false-positive rate of EFM for predicting adverse outcomes is high. The use of EFM is associated with an increase in the rate of operative interventions (vacuum, forceps, and cesarean delivery)."[3] Other factors causing cesarean deliveries to grow include the unwillingness of physicians to give women who had previous cesarean sections a trial of labor before resorting to the procedure, the diminished education of residents in the non-surgical delivery of babies who occupy a breech presentation in the womb,[4] and the growing number of women who either become pregnant at an older age and at higher-than-average risk for having birth complications or who opt for early delivery for personal considerations. But the increased risks to babies born before term revealed by a 2009 study is likely to curtail this latter option.[5]

The widespread use of a questionably effective technology such as EFM, and a retreat from using alternative nonsurgical interventions to deliver growing numbers of babies also is influenced in America by a legal factor. As a 1989 National Academy of Sciences study noted, it is the "physicians' perception that the majority of allegations in obstetric suits involve the issues of fetal monitoring and failure to perform timely cesarean section."[6] Lent in a 1999 *Stanford Law Review* article argues against this perception: "Legal analysis," she writes, "reveals that the law is on the side of obstetricians who provide their patients with the best care, including safer, more effective methods of monitoring fetal heartrate during labor and delivery. Employment of the EFM technique fails to further this objective. Instead, it jeopardizes outcomes for both mothers and infants by causing unnecessary interventions."[7] While legal pressures influence a doctor's decision making, Lent notes, "The reverse is true to a far greater degree. Physicians' decisions influence medicolegal pressure." The law grants to the medical profession the prerogative to establish what standards of care are best for patients. Accordingly, the profession has the duty as well as the ability to soundly evaluate the technologies that practitioners apply to avoid their unwise and ineffective use. In taking such steps, physicians can help "remove 'defensive medicine' as a priority consideration in medical decision making."[8] Finally, it should be noted that choosing technological measures as the primary means to implement defensive practice in obstetrics and in other areas of medicine demonstrates their hold on medical thinking and practice.

References:
1. Sachs BP. Is the Rising Rate of Cesarean Sections a Result of More Defensive Medicine? In *Medical Professional Liability and the Delivery of Obstetric Care: Volume II, An Interdisciplinary Review*. Washington, D.C.: National Academy of Sciences; 1989, 28; CDC Reports. Available at: http://aww.cdc.gov/hch9/pressroom/o1facts/cesarian.htm; Tita ATN, Landon, MR, Spring CY, et al. Timing of Elective Repeat Cesarean Delivery at Term and Neonatal Outcomes. *New England Journal of Medicine*. 2009; 360(2):11120. 2. Intrapartum Fetal Heart Rate Monitoring. *ACOG Practice Bulletin*. 2005; 70:1. 3. Ibid., 7. 4. Sachs, op. cit., 32. 5. Tita ATN, Landon, MR, Spring CY, et al., op. cit., 6. Sachs, op. cit., 38. 7. Lent M. The Medical and Legal Risks of the Electronic Fetal Monitor. *Stanford Law Review*. 1999; 51(4):836. 8. Ibid., 837. The term defensive medicine describes clinical actions taken by physicians in part to avoid potential legal risks.
43. Martell LK. From Innovation to Common Practice: Prenatal Nursing Pre-1970–2005. *Journal of Perinatal Neonatal Nursing*. 2006; 20(1):8–16.
44. National Center for Health Statistics, op. cit.

CHAPTER 9. GOVERNING THE EMPIRE OF MACHINES

1. Jones WHS (trans.). *The Oath*. In *Hippocrates*. Cambridge, Mass.: Harvard University Press; 1962, 164–5.
2. *Decorum*. In ibid., 319.
3. Oken D. What to Tell Cancer Patients: A Study of Medical Attitudes. *JAMA*. 1961; 175:1120–8.
4. Waitzken H, Stoeckle JD. The Communication of Information about Illness. *Advances in Psychosomatic Medicine*. 1972; 8:185–9.
5. American Hospital Association. Statement on a Patient's Bill of Rights. *Hospitals*. 1973; 47:41.
6. Reiser SJ. Words as Scalpels: Transmitting Evidence in the Clinical Dialogue. *Annals of Internal Medicine*. 1980; 92:837–42.
7. Personal communication: Stephen Greenberg, History of Medicine Division, National Library of Medicine, Bethesda, Md., Aug. 2008.
8. Riessman F, Carroll D. *Redefining Self-Help Policy and Practice*. San Francisco: Jossey-Bass Publishers; 1995, 3.
9. *The New York Times Guide to Essential Knowledge*. New York: St. Martin's Press; 2004, 654.
10. Ferguson T. *Health Online*. Reading, Mass.: Addison-Wesley Publishing; 1996, xix.
11. McNay MB, Fleming JEE. Forty Years of Obstetric Ultrasound 1957–1997: From A-Scope to Three Dimensions. *Ultrasound in Medicine and Biology*. 1999; 25(1):4–5.
12. Ibid., 8–11. For most of recorded history, the state of the living human fetus was known best to pregnant women. They felt and described body changes at first appreciated only by them and shared with others through choice and special relationships. Technologies that permitted practitioners to detect signs of pregnancy, which the woman who carried the fetus could not dependably monitor, began with a nonvisual technology. In 1822 the French physician

de Kergaradec found that the detection and evaluation of fetal heart sounds could be accomplished with the stethoscope, thus allowing physicians to learn whether the fetus was alive or dead.[1] But the sounds could not be discerned until after the fifth month of pregnancy. Enter the X-ray, which, from its invention at the end of the nineteenth century, was applied routinely to follow fetal development. Its expert medical users failed in this as in other areas of medicine to appreciate its risks to the examined and the examiner, and they believed its benefits outweighed growing warnings of danger. X-ray imaging captivated obstetric doctors with its ability to gauge fetal age and detect fetal disease such as the serious neurological disorder spina bifida, to distinguish pregnancy from other sources of an enlarging abdomen such as tumors, and even to display the early existence of pregnancy itself. In 1930 an obstetrician wrote: "Antenatal work without the routine use of X-rays is no more justifiable than would be the treatment of fractures."[2] The dangers of radiation revealed in the 1940s and 1950s essentially ended the routine use of X-rays in obstetrics and closed the visual path through which to chart fetal development. But it reopened rather soon, lit by a new agent of imaging.

References:
1. de Kergaradec JAL. Mémoire sur l'auscultation appliquée à l'étude de la grosse. Paris; 1822. 2. Oakley A. *The Captured Womb: A History of the Medical Care of Pregnant Women.* Oxford, U.K.: Basil Blackwell; 1990, 103.
13. A 1980 Consensus Conference report declared its general safety, but it cautioned doctors that only explicit medical indications should lead to ultrasound examinations. Still, belief in their safety and significance overcame misgivings by physicians about their potential and unknown harms. By the 1990s many doctors offered ultrasound scans to mothers wanting to see their fetus, a reassurance that seemed a significant benefit to doctor and patient, particularly if prior problems with pregnancy existed. McNay and Fleming, op. cit, 8–11, 34. See also Goldberg BB. Obstetric U.S. Imaging: The Past 40 Years. *Radiology.* 2000; 215:622–9.
14. McNay and Fleming, op. cit., 27–49.
15. Ibid., 49–50.
16. Rothman BK. *The Tentative Pregnancy: Prenatal Diagnosis and the Future of Motherhood.* New York: Viking; 1986, 113–14.
17. Petchesky RP. Foetal Images: The Power of Visual Culture in the Politics of Reproduction. In Stamworth M (ed.), *Reproductive Technologies: Gender, Motherhood, and Medicine.* Minneapolis: University of Minnesota Press; 1987, 64.
18. Saetman AR. Thirteen Women's Narratives of Pregnancy, Ultrasound, and Self. In Saetman AR, Oudshoorn N, Kirejczyk M (eds.), *Bodies of Technology: Women's Involvement with Reproductive Medicine.* Columbus: Ohio State University Press; 2000, 340–1. See also Holmqvist T. *The Hospital Is a Uterus: Western Discourses of Childbirth in Late Modernity – A Case Study from Northern Italy.* Stockholm: Studies in Social Anthropology; 2000, 118–19.

19. Saetman, op. cit., 306–7.
20. Parker-Pope T. Doctor and Patient, Now at Odds. *New York Times*, July 29, 2008, D6.
21. Dubos RJ. *Man Adapting.* New Haven, Conn.: Yale University Press; 1965, xviii–xix.

INDEX

Morgagni, G. B., 4, 137–138, 186
mortality reduction, 177–178
Morton, William T. G., 169–172
Mountain Electric Company, 23
multiphasic population screening, 146–148

narrative. *See* patient's narrative/
  perspective
National Academy of Sciences' Institute of
  Medicine, 96
National Foundation for Infantile
  Paralysis, 59
National Health Council, 142–143
National Institutes of Health, 48–49
Natural Death Act, 71
Necheles, Heinrich, 33
negative pressure devices, 52, 53. *See also*
  artificial respirators/respiration
The New England Journal of Medicine,
  78–79
New Jersey Supreme Court, 65, 66–69
*A New Perspective on the Health of
  Canadians* (Lalonde), 152–153
Nightingale, Florence, 76
*Nosologia methodica, sistems morborum
  classes, genera et species* (de
  Sauvages), 136
numerical method, in treatment evaluation,
  110–111

Obama, Barack, 98
objectivity. *See also* patient's
  narrative/perspective
  in depiction of illness, 27–29
  elimination of subjective elements, 29–30
  of medical findings, 26
  of photography/X-rays, 26–29
observer bias, 113–115
observer variance, 19, 28
obstetric forceps
  concealment of, 158, 164
  origins/use of, 162–169
"On a New Kind of Rays, A Preliminary
  Communication" (Röntgen), 21
Oregon Basic Health Services Act, 121–128
"Osmotic Force" (Graham), 32
Our Bodies, Ourselves (Boston Women's
  Health Book Collective), 183–184
Outdoor Department (New York Lying-In
  Hospital), 178–180

Pasteur, Louis, 175–177
pathology
  clinical-pathological conferences, 77–79
  study of, 4
patient record
  adequacy of, 83–84
  computerization of, 90–92, 96
  costs of, 103
  in doctor's head, 84–85
  electronic health record (EHR), 96–99
  End Result System, 80–82
  ethical/legal dimensions, 102
    follow-up system, 82–83
  and government/social oversight, 94–96
  HIPPA legislation, 101–102
  hospital standards/record keeping, 79,
    85–86
  in medical education, 77–79
  and Medicare/Medicaid, 95
  mission of, 74
  multiple use fulfillment, 102–103
  19th century development of, 74–77,
    103
  personal health record, 100–101
  PROMIS, 92–94
  and quality of care, 79
  and specialization, 85
  standardization, 87–90
  telecommunications, use of, 94
  unified records, 86–87
  unifying role, 103–104
Patient's Bill of Rights, 191
patient's narrative/perspective
  and diagnostic technologies, 12–13
  in early works of medicine, 1–3
  rejection/disregard of, 26, 27
  truth of personal meaning, 29
Pearl, Raymond, 87–89
Pearson, Karl, 27
pectoriloquism, 7
Peebles, Allen, 84–85
Percival, Thomas, 171–172
periodic medical examination, 140–145
personal health record, 100–101. *See also*
  patient record
Petchesky, R. P., 199
Peterson, Osler, 84–85
photography, 18–20, 26–28
phthisis. *See* tuberculosis
physical examination. *See also* periodic
    medical examination
  doctors' restraint in, 3
  and modesty/privacy, 4–5
  periodic, 140–145
  vs. technological examination, 24–25,
    29
The Physician (Hippocrates), 132
Physician Standards Review Organizations,
  95
physicians
  and medical technology limits, 71–72
  medication information disclosure,
    189–193
  and periodic examinations, 143–145
Pintard, John, 151–152

Supportive Care Protocol, 71–72
surgery/surgeons, 9–10, 23
Swedish Hospital of Seattle, 42–43
Sydenham, Thomas, 133–137, 138, 186
Symcotts, John, 2
symptoms
  categories of, 134
  and concept of disease, 135–137
syphilis, screening for, 146
systematic research reviews, 120–121

"technological breakthroughs," 1
technology
  absorptive/reflective nature of, 186–188
  advocacy of new, 29–30
  influence on patient care, 50–51
  limits on use, 70–72
  nature of, 51
  relation to humanism, 188–189,
    201–203
  spending on, 51
telecommunications, use of, 94. *See also*
  patient record
Teschan, Paul E., 40
Thalhimer, William, 33–34
Thank You, Dr. Lamaze (Karmel),
  184–185
"They Decide Who Lives, Who Dies"
  (Alexander), 44–46
transplantation
  ethics and, 63–65
  of kidneys, 41–42
  and Oregon Basic Health Services Act,
    121–122
*Treatise on Diseases of the Chest, and on
  Mediate Auscultation* (Laennec), 7–8
treatment evaluation, numerical method in,
  110–111
tuberculosis, 7, 18–19, 134–135
Turner, B., 32–33
2001: A Space Odyssey, 199

ultrasound technology, 194–200
unified record, 86–87. *See also* patient
  record
unions, and worker health, 141

Van Helmont, Jean Baptiste, 111
Van Leeuwenhoek, Antoni, 18
Van Noordwijk, Jakob, 36
ventilators, 53. *See also* artificial
  respirators/respiration
Vesalius, Andreas, 4, 14–15, 52–53, 137
Veterans Administration, 48–49
Virchow, Rudolph, 139

Waitzkin, H., 190–191
Waksman, Selman, 117
Wald, Lillian, 140
Walter Reed Army Hospital, 48
Warren, John Collins, 169–172
Wasserman test, 146
Web-based information system, 97
Weed, Lawrence, 92–94
Wilbanks, E. R., 166–167
Williams, Francis, 24
Wilson, J. L., 54–55
Winterscheld, Loren, 41
women's health movement, 181–184
workplace
  period medical examination in, 141
  physical handicaps in, 150
World Health Organization (WHO),
  152–153
World War I, and national fitness, 129,
  142
World War II
  artificial kidney creation, 31–32
  radiation danger awareness, 24
  X-ray interpretation, 28
Wright, James Homer, 77–79

X-ray
  diagnostic reliance on, 24–25
  discovery/invention of, 20–21
  health damage/radiation dangers, 23–24
  objectivity/authenticity of, 26–29
  in obstetrics, 221
  public/professional reaction to, 21–23
  as screening agent, 145–146
  vs. stethoscope, 26

Young, James, 180

Printed in the United States
By Bookmasters